WWFD (What Would Florence Do?)

WWFD
(What Would Florence Do?)

A Guide for New Nurse Managers

Sue Johnson, PhD, RN, NE-BC

American Nurses Association
Silver Spring, Maryland • 2015

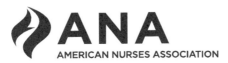

ANA
AMERICAN NURSES ASSOCIATION

American Nurses Association
8515 Georgia Avenue, Suite 400
Silver Spring, MD 20910-3492
1-800-274-4ANA
www.NursingWorld.org

The American Nurses Association (ANA) is the premier organization representing the interests of the nation's 3.6 million registered nurses. ANA advances the nursing profession by fostering high standards of nursing practice, promoting a safe and ethical work environment, bolstering the health and wellness of nurses, and advocating on health care issues that affect nurses and the public. ANA is at the forefront of improving the quality of health care for all.

Library of Congress Cataloging-in-Publication Data

Johnson, Sue (Carol Susan), 1946-, author.
  WWFD (what would Florence do?): a guide for new nurse managers / Sue Johnson.
      p. ; cm.
  Includes bibliographical references and index.
  Summary: "A guide for new nurse managers, with Florence Nightingale as a mentor. Includes Nightingale-based perspectives on advocacy, communication, conflict and collaboration, career and staff development, community partnerships, evidence- and research-based practice, resource and fiscal management, safety, and strategic planning in health care and nursing"—Provided by publisher.
  ISBN 978-1-55810-583-6 (alk. paper) — ISBN 978-1-55810-584-3 — ISBN 978-1-55810-585-0 — ISBN 978-1-55810-586-7
  I. Title.
  [DNLM: 1. Nursing Care—organization & administration. 2. Nursing, Supervisory. WY 105]
  RT51
  610.73—dc23
                                    2014043008

978-1-55810-583-6   SAN: 851-3481   02/2017R
 First printing: December 2014.   Second printing: November 2015.
Third printing: February 2017

To my parents, Charles L. and Margaret M. Johnson,
whose love and support always encouraged me
to seek excellence in nursing and in life.

Contents

Introduction

Congratulations!

You've just accepted your first nurse manager position. Whether the title is nurse manager, nurse leader, or team leader, you are accountable for the success or failure of your unit, your team, and even your organization. That is a tremendous responsibility and an awesome opportunity. You have a right to be nervous about learning a new role and honing the leadership skills you will now use on a daily basis. It's no longer enough to be a proficient staff nurse. Your new nursing world is strange, challenging, and fascinating. However, you know you will need education and support to develop into a transformational nurse leader. Manager orientation will give you lots of useful information about staffing, budgeting, communicating, evaluating, and project management. An experienced nurse manager mentor will also reduce your learning curve. If you have difficulty finding such a mentor, here is an introduction to a transformational nurse mentor who can help you make those difficult decisions: Florence Nightingale.

Most nurses today only think of Florence Nightingale as "The Lady with the Lamp" in Scutari during the Crimean War (Nightingale, 1992). That is only a small aspect of her numerous accomplishments—accomplishments that influence the future of our profession during this era of healthcare reform. As new nurse managers who must navigate current regulatory, quality, and reimbursement issues, it is time for each of us to ask "WWFD (What Would Florence Do)?" The answers will surprise you and guide you as a nurse manager into a nursing future that benefits both nurses, patients, and our profession.

A Perspective About Health Care Today

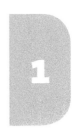

Regulatory, quality, and reimbursement issues reflect the complexity of our current healthcare environment. Hospitals' ability to manage their bottom line is affected by all these forces. The Affordable Care Act established the Hospital Value-Based Purchasing Program (Centers for Medicare and Medicaid Services, 2013b), which began providing incentive payments to hospitals based on quality, not quantity, of care provided to Medicare patients beginning at the start of Fiscal Year (FY) 2013. This potential for additional reimbursement puts hospitals at risk for reimbursement reduction (1.0% of base operating Diagnosis Related Group amounts in Fiscal Year (FY) 2013 and 2.0% by Fiscal Year (FY) 2017) if they fail to meet clinical process of care measures (70%) and patient experience of care measures (30%). The impact of empowered nurses on the hospital's bottom line is as great today as the impact of Florence Nightingale on healthcare reform in the formative years of our profession. Let's take a closer look at the parallels between the two as we get acquainted with Florence and her achievements.

Florence and the Nurse Manager

Florence's contributions to health care included emphasis on quality patient-centered care based on the best available evidence. To achieve this quality patient care, she knew that nurses had to be educated and observant to make wise judgments that promoted the health of their patients (Nightingale, 1992). The 2011 Institute of Medicine Report echoes Florence's message that nurses should practice fully based on their training and education and should be full partners with physicians and other healthcare professionals in healthcare redesign (Institute of Medicine, 2011). Staff nurses, in their daily work, influence many of the clinical processes of care and patient experience of care measures in the Value-Based Purchasing (VBP) Program. Perioperative and Surgical unit nurses are experts on clinical SCIP measures, such as prophylactic antibiotic use, Beta Blocker administration, controlled postoperative serum glucose in cardiac patients, and Venous Thromboembolism (VTE) prophylaxis. In FY 2014, the Value-Based Purchasing Program will also require post-operative urinary catheter removal on post-operative day 1 or 2 (Centers for Medicare and Medicaid Services, 2013b). Staff nurses will play an integral role in the success or failure of this additional clinical process of care measure and sound leadership, but nurse managers must support staff nurses in achieving the goals of the Value-Based Purchasing Program and Hospital Consumer Assessment of Healthcare Providers and Systems (HCAHPS). HCAHPS is a national survey that asks recent patients about their experience during their hospital stay. These results are posted nationally to compare hospitals based on ten important hospital quality topics (Centers for Medicare and Medicaid Services, 2013a).

Since 30% of Value-Based Purchasing reimbursement is based on patient experience of care measures, HCAHPS scores gauge how well, or poorly, the patient rates his or her experience (Centers for Medicare and Medicaid Services, 2013a). Florence understood how important it is for staff nurses to spend time getting to know their patients and communicating with them. In her *Notes on Nursing,* she emphasized the importance of informing the patient when the nurse will be returning, listening to the patient's concerns, observing the patient for condition changes, reducing unnecessary noise, ensuring confidentiality and privacy, and using appropriate infection control measures, especially hand hygiene (Nightingale, 1992). These measures are as important in today's hospitals as they were in Florence's time, and leadership by nurse managers and staff nurses in each of these measures can result in higher patient ratings of their hospital experience. These higher ratings can positively influence the hospitals' Value-Based Purchasing reimbursement. Providing the opportunity for nurses to interact and know their patients beyond just the disease process is priceless.

The Nurse Manager's Role

Florence described the role of the charge nurse as not only carrying out nursing skills and duties, but also ensuring that everyone else follows proper procedures in patient care in the charge nurse's absence (Nightingale, 1992). Substitute 'nurse manager' for 'charge nurse' and her statement is applicable to today's nursing culture. It is your responsibility to ensure that patients receive timely, efficient, effective, and patient-focused care. Florence was a lifelong proponent of healthcare reform. She used statistical data to support the reforms she advocated and was the first person to recognize the need for uniform hospital statistics throughout the world (Nightingale, 1992). As a nurse manager today, you need to pay careful attention to unit and hospital statistics that include nurse-sensitive indicators, i.e. "processes and outcomes that are affected, provided, and/or influenced by nursing personnel, but for which nursing is not exclusively responsible" (National Quality Forum, p. 2). These indicators include:

- Nursing hours per patient day (NHPPD)
- Nursing skill mix
- Nurse turnover rate
- RN education/certification
- NDNQI RN satisfaction survey results
- Catheter-associated urinary tract infection rates
- Central line-associated blood stream infection rates
- Fall/injury fall rates
- Hospital/unit acquired pressure ulcer rates
- Pain assessment/intervention/reassessment cycles
- Peripheral IV infiltration rates
- Physical restraint prevalence
- Ventilator-associated pneumonia rates (American Nurses Association, 2013b).

You must carefully evaluate these indicators for trends and note improvements resulting from the nurses' roles in providing quality patient-centered care. You also must share this information with unit staff members and organization leaders. It is imperative for you to provide a therapeutic climate in the unit for unit staff members, other healthcare team members, and patients/families. You must also advocate for resources that will enable staff nurses to spend quality time interacting with patients and families and ensure that this interaction occurs consistently.

Florence had significant influence on the British Empire in improving health and sanitation of hospitals as well as on the development of professional nursing. She collaborated with elected leaders, bureaucrats, and even Queen Victoria on healthcare issues of her day (Nightingale, 1992). Like Florence, you and other nurse managers are organization decision-makers and are in a unique position to promote the achievements of your staff nurses in nurse-sensitive indicators that impact the hospital's bottom line. Nurses have an exceptional opportunity to influence their organizations as Value-Based Purchasing is implemented nationally. You and other nurse managers collaborate with leaders of many hospital departments on a daily basis. You must share the success stories of your nursing staff in meeting Value-Based Purchasing requirements, nurse-sensitive indicators, and the impact these successes have on the organization's bottom line. You are responsible to advocate for unit-based resources that will advance the organization's mission and the future of nursing in the organization.

Just as Florence devoted her life to her mission, you must devote time and energy to the mission of the organization and the nursing department. As Florence encouraged nurses to collect empirical data about patients' conditions to make wise judgments about care delivery (Nightingale, 1992), you must use empirical data for the same purpose. Since Florence aligned herself with influential leaders to facilitate healthcare changes (Nightingale, 1992), you must also align with influential organization leaders, such as the CFO, to meet the regulatory, quality, and reimbursement challenges of 2013 and beyond.

The Future of Health Care

This is a pivotal time for nurses to assume leadership roles in health care. As a nurse manager, you owe it to yourself, your patients, and your profession to stay educated and informed about changes in healthcare reform. Don't hesitate to make your voice heard in decision-making that will impact your practice. Ask yourself "WWFD—What Would Florence Do?" The answer will affect how well you navigate healthcare reform and influence the future of nursing. The future of health care will provide significant opportunities for nurses to validate Florence Nightingale's statements about nursing in disease and wellness. "[T]here is universal experience as to the extreme importance of careful nursing in determining the issue of the disease. The same laws of health or of nursing, for they are in reality the same, obtain among the well as among the sick" (Nightingale 1992, p. 6). Although the wording is from a different era, Florence's message echoes that of the 2011 Institute of Medicine's vision of "... a practice environment that is fundamentally transformed so that nurses are efficiently employed—whether in the hospital or in the community—to the full extent of their education, skills, and competencies" (Institute of Medicine, p. 30). The future will require skilled, capable nurses who will lead their organizations and profession to the truly patient-focused care envisioned by Florence Nightingale in the 1800s.

Strategic Planners

2

Florence's Role

Transformational leaders are experts at strategic planning (American Nurses Credentialing Center, 2008), and Florence Nightingale was a transformational nurse leader. This was evident in her first nursing leadership position. In 1851, Florence was 30 years old and had completed a three-month training course for nurses at the hospital in Kaiserwerth, Germany. Her Kaiserwerth experience enabled Florence to understand the basic components of nursing care, hospital design, and personnel administration. That year was pivotal in her life and in the future of nursing as a profession. Two years later, Florence was hired as Superintendent of the Hospital for Gentlewomen in Distressed Circumstances at number one Harley Street in central London. The small private hospital was a facility in poor condition with an inadequately trained staff. Five patients died in the first month of occupancy, and Florence had to contend with a gas leak resulting in a series of small explosions, a drunken supervisor, and a fight between workmen. Her first nursing leadership position also gave Florence an opportunity to engage in strategic planning to improve the hospital's efficiency and effectiveness. She had the support of the Ladies' Committee to whom she reported her strategic planning. This resulted in the creation and implementation of environmental and patient care standards to improve the hospital course for all patients. Florence's nursing vision—that all patients deserved competent care by qualified nurses—became a reality during her twelve months as Superintendent (Selanders, Lake, & Crane, 2010). Her emphasis on strategic planning continued in Scutari and in development of the Nightingale School at St. Thomas' Hospital in London after the Crimean War (Baly, 1986).

The Nurse Manager's Role

Today, nurse managers play a significant role in strategic planning for their units and their organization. You are accountable and responsible for the safe provision of patient care on the unit. You play an integral role in strategic planning by ensuring that care delivery on the unit supports the nursing and organization strategic plans (American Nurses Credentialing Center, 2008). You must clearly understand strategic priorities as Florence did and communicate them to unit staff members. This dialogue is an opportunity for you to elicit support for current and anticipated strategic priorities. Your role is pivotal in improving unit effectiveness and efficiency by clinical expertise and sound communication with the nursing staff members to initiate changes to better address strategic priorities. As Florence honed her leadership skills during her year on Harley Street, you must continuously hone your leadership skills to articulate resource needs and develop the knowledge and skills of unit staff members. It is vital that staff members work as a team to support positive patient care outcomes in accordance with organization and nursing strategic and quality plans (American Nurses Credentialing Center, 2008). To address strategic and quality initiatives, the leadership role of the nurse manager must include zero tolerance for disruptive behavior and an emphasis on teamwork and collaboration.

Staff nurses must be able to articulate how the nursing mission, vision, values, and strategic and quality plans relate to the organization's strategic priorities (American Nurses Credentialing Center, 2008). Based on Florence's vision of provision of competent care by qualified nurses, they must also know how their unit and their activities support the organization's strategic plan. If the organization's strategic priority for the coming fiscal year is to reduce readmissions within thirty days for patients with congestive heart failure, the staff nurses on the Telemetry unit must ensure that these patients are educated about how to care for themselves at home, including diet, activity, medications, and follow-up (Centers for Medicare and Medicaid Services, 2013b). The staff nurse's role is vital to the success of this strategic initiative, and the nurse manager must ensure that staff nurses are knowledgeable about both hospital and nursing strategic and quality plans and their part in the success of these plans. This is not a one-time discussion for a unit meeting. The hospital and nursing mission, vision, values, and strategic and quality plans are not just empty words on annual reports. They include structures, processes, and expectations to improve the organization's effectiveness and efficiency (American Nurses Credentialing Center, 2008).

The nurse manager's leadership and influence on the unit team mirrors that of Florence as Superintendent of the small private hospital in London. As Florence emphasized strategic planning throughout her career, the nurse manager plays an integral role in strategic planning to improve effectiveness and efficiency on the unit by ensuring competent care by qualified nurses. If the hospital and nursing strategic priority is enhancing ED throughput, the nurse manager must confirm that appropriate resources are on the unit to facilitate patients' admission and care during each shift (Centers for Medicare and Medicaid Services, 2013a). Using input from staff nurses, the nurse manager advocates for resources to safeguard care delivery during all shifts. These resources may include additional staff members to meet patient needs, technology resources to ensure comprehensive documentation of treatment and clinical issues, or housekeeping support to ensure a clean, safe patient environment. Florence's emphasis on the hospital environment plays a key role in the nurse manager's interactions with housekeeping personnel as we want to ensure a timely response to room preparation. This is an essential component in meeting this strategic goal. The nurse manager must also serve as the voice of staff nurses to organizational leaders. You must regularly seek staff input about environmental and patient care issues that may affect unit performance in meeting nursing and organizational strategic priorities. As Florence used statistical data to advocate for improved patient care standards, today's nurse manager must use statistical data from multiple data sources to determine the staffing requirements needed to achieve strategic goals. If a strategic goal for the coming year is to increase patient volume by implementation of a new service on the unit (e.g. implementation of a transfusion clinic on the Oncology unit), the nurse manager is responsible and accountable for ensuring safe staffing levels and clinical knowledge to care for these patients (American Nurses Credentialing Center, 2008). Often, adjustments to unit staffing levels require negotiation between the nurse manager and professional colleagues about resource allocation to achieve the strategic goal.

Your own education fuels your participation in strategic planning on the unit and within the organization. As a new nurse manager, you must develop a sound understanding of the hospital and nursing mission, vision, and values as well as determine how you will integrate these into the daily activities of your unit. Pay close attention when the strategic and quality plans are discussed in orientation classes and management meetings. Don't be afraid to seek the guidance of your nurse leader or CNO if you have questions about the expectations for your unit and staff members. Florence used the support of the Ladies' Committee to improve the hospital's care delivery system based on her strategic planning. New nurse managers should use the support of their leaders to achieve positive outcomes based on their facility and nursing's strategic planning processes.

Commitment to Nursing

3

Florence's Role

Nursing as a Career Choice

Florence Nightingale's choice of nursing as her vocation began in her childhood. Born the second of two daughters of a prosperous English family, Florence nursed and bandaged the dolls her older sister damaged (Cook, 1913a). As a child, she also gave first aid to save a collie with a broken leg and wrote a prescription in a small book (Cook, 1913a). What made Florence unique, however, was her sense of a "calling" and dedication to a life in the service of God at the age of sixteen on February 7, 1837 (Cook, 1913a). At seventeen, Florence and her family journeyed to Italy and France for what became a two-year tour (September 8, 1837–April 6, 1839) (Cook, 1913a). During this time, an English lady in the hotel where Florence and her family stayed in Italy became ill and Florence volunteered to nurse her to her subsequent recovery (Cook, 1913a). In the winter of 1838–39, the Nightingale family was in Paris and the city's hospitals and nursing sisterhoods fascinated Florence (Cook, 1913a). On her return home, Florence became the go-to person of her family in dealing with illness. In 1845, she nursed her paternal grandmother into partial recovery and cared for her old nurse, Gale, in her last illness (Cook, 1913a). As her sense of vocation increased, Florence wanted to go to Salisbury Hospital later that year to study nursing, but her mother would not permit it (Cook, 1913a). At the time, there were moral and social objections to nursing, and many nurses were drunks and women of questionable character. That a refined and genteel lady like Florence Nightingale would consider becoming a nurse was unthinkable in her society (Cook, 1913a). Florence was nothing if not persistent and she finally achieved her goal (Cook, 1913a).

Commitment to Nursing

Her commitment to nursing never wavered. In 1853, she left her holiday early to help admit and care for women cholera patients at Middlesex Hospital, where she was not employed (Cook, 1913a). In the Crimea, Florence epitomized the compassionate and caring nurse by going the extra mile to support dying patients (Cook, 1913a). She believed that service to man also served God, thus her main desire was to raise nursing to a trained calling. Florence believed that nurses should be devoted to their calling and organized on a secular basis (Cook, 1913a). She was concerned with complacency and considered nursing a vocation and art that required constant study (Selanders & Crane, 2012; Cook, 1913b). Florence's philosophy held that nurses must always make progress and gain experience to serve God through the highest level of service to man (Cook, 1913b). Even though she valued efficiency, Florence wanted her nurses to focus on compassion for the sick and desire to serve others (Cook, 1913b). In 1893, Florence contributed a paper to a Congress on women's work in Chicago that exemplified her commitment to nursing: "A new art, and a new science, has been created since and within the last forty years. And with it a new profession—so they say; we say *calling*." (Cook, 1913b, p. 365)

The Nurse Manager's Role

Nursing as a Career Choice

Why did you become a nurse? This is a vital question for you to answer because the answer will affect how you focus your efforts as a new nurse manager. Once you clearly understand your own motivation, as Florence did, then you can guide your nursing staff to best address patients' needs and their own professional growth. "A philosophy is a statement of the central beliefs and values that direct decisions and activities" (Grif-Alspach, 1995, p. 4). Think of your philosophy as the framework that will direct your daily activities.

Try a fun exercise to develop **your** personal nursing philosophy:

1. Take an 8x11 piece of paper and draw a line down the middle.
2. List five beliefs you hold about nursing as a profession on the left side.

3. Next to each belief, write a few words about how you can make that belief a reality in your new role.

4. Now, use this information to write a paragraph or two (no more) that will represent your personal nursing philosophy.

5. Review the philosophy of your organization and the nursing department and compare your personal nursing philosophy with both documents. You will be surprised to find how well they complement each other.

6. Share your nursing philosophy with your team and encourage them to develop their own nursing philosophy.

7. Laminate your philosophy and post it on your overhead so you can refer to it at regular intervals.

8. When you review your nursing philosophy, change and update it as needed so it is always current, timely, and congruent with your organization and department philosophy statements and needs (Grif-Alspach, 1995).

Some of you always wanted to be a nurse as Florence did. Others may have tried other career avenues before deciding that nursing was the best choice for you. Nursing is a profession that includes multiple areas of practice. You have been chosen as nursing manager for your clinical area. Now, it is up to you to put your nursing philosophy into practice to benefit your patients, staff, unit, and organization.

Commitment to Nursing

Florence demonstrated her commitment to nursing throughout her life. You will have a steep learning curve as you become a nurse manager, but managerial skills are not sufficient. You also need to continue to focus on honing your nursing skills and knowledge. You are in a profession that cares for people at traumatic times in their lives. Technical skill is only one aspect of nursing practice. You have assumed a role of accountability and responsibility. It is now up to you to ensure that your unit's focus on patient care is tempered by compassion, caring, and empathy. You have a unique opportunity to put your nursing philosophy into practice and to develop your nursing team members. Encourage them to use evidence and continue to develop their nursing and people skills. That will only happen if you demonstrate your own commitment to your profession. Florence was a pioneer in the reform of nursing (Selanders & Crane, 2012). Now, it is your turn to move nursing forward in the 21st century. You are a role model for both patients and staff in your daily activities. As a nurse manager, your values are important and must be visible in your interactions. It is time to take your nursing philosophy to reality in your new role. You, your staff members, and most of all, your patients will benefit from your commitment to nursing (American Nurses Association, 2009).

The Journey to Healthcare Advocacy

4

Florence's Role

Advocacy requires courage of convictions and Florence Nightingale always displayed the courage of her convictions. When she accepted the position of Superintendent at the Hospital for Gentlewomen in Distressed Circumstances, she was a novice nurse leader who was not afraid to challenge the status quo. The Ladies' Committee determined that only members of the Church of England could be admitted and receive treatment at the Hospital. Florence was raised as a liberal Unitarian. She believed every individual was valuable regardless of religious preference. This difference in philosophy caused Florence to threaten to leave the position if it could not be resolved. When the Committee realized that she was serious about advocating for patients of all religions as well as agnostics and atheists, they reconsidered their decision and agreed with her approach. This was the beginning of Florence's role as a healthcare advocate (Selanders & Crane, 2012).

Nurse Advocacy

Florence's advocacy for nurses was evident in her appointment as Superintendent of Nurses in the Crimean War of 1854. In November of that year, Florence arrived in what is now Turkey with 38 handpicked nurses of various backgrounds and experience. She had an official appointment from

Sidney Herbert, British Secretary for War, to supervise nursing care under the direction of the Chief Army Medical Officer of Hospitals at Scutari, a suburb of Constantinople. The Barrack Hospital was filled with wounded and dying soldiers and conditions were deplorable. Florence knew that her nurses faced resentment by some of the medical officers who saw no need for women in the war zone. She ensured that they cared only for patients with surgeons' permission while she did night rounds herself so they could return to their quarters at a reasonable hour. The nurses' quarters were cramped and infected with vermin. Nurses became ill with fevers and Florence advocated for them by using her own money to pay for a house in Scutari for ill nurses to recover (Cook, 1913a). After her return home, Florence advocated for nursing education and nursing expansion outside hospital walls to meet growing healthcare needs. She advocated for the nurse's role in managing the patient's environment and encouraged nurses to be patient advocates (Selanders & Crane, 2012).

Patient Advocacy

Florence was a tireless advocate for patients throughout her lifetime. In Scutari, she focused on improving the environment of care for wounded soldiers. Besides focusing on cleanliness and efficiency, Florence pushed against stoppages of soldiers' pay when they were sick. She focused on the moral and mental well-being of these soldiers and encouraged them to send part of their pay home to their families. She fought for a Government Store House for goods and provisions and became the Purveyor-Auxiliary to provide essential supplies to the hospitals (Cook, 1913a). She continued her advocacy after the War, by persistent lobbying for the health of the military and the people of India (Cook, 1913a). Her *Notes on Nursing* illustrates Florence's holistic view of how nurses' advocacy for patients is demonstrated by attention to environmental factors and focus on prevention (Nightingale, 1992).

The Role of Nursing

Florence's advocacy was particularly evident in her support for improving the qualifications of nurses. Nurses who graduated from the Nightingale Training School for Nurses were widely sought as lady superintendents (Cook, 1913b). The result of her advocacy was the introduction into British hospitals of an organized system of trained nursing (Cook, 1913b).

The Nurse Manager's Role

As a nurse manager, you know that change is constant in health care today. Successful change will require you to advocate for your patients, your staff members, and the role of nursing in your facility. It is your responsibility to guide the evolution of both planned and unplanned change (American Nurses Credentialing Center, 2008). In your role, you must serve as a patient advocate on a daily basis to navigate such changes in the patients' best interest. Let's explore a couple of scenarios that demonstrate how you can advocate for patients during changes—both planned and unplanned.

Patient Advocacy

Here is an example of how you can be a patient advocate by facilitating a planned change. When you round on surgical patients, you hear frequent complaints about inability to rest. Their concerns reflect Florence's in *Notes on Nursing*: "Unnecessary noise, then, is the most cruel absence of care which can be inflicted either on sick or well" (Nightingale, 1992, p. 27). Since adequate rest facilitates healing, you discuss this issue at staff meetings to explore possible changes. A volunteer from each shift assesses noise levels at different times of the day, and other team members review the literature for alternatives. Noise levels at night are higher than they should be and you advocate lowering the decibels so patients can better rest (Murphy, Bernardo, & Dalton, 2013). You also explore literature about having a rest period—'nap time'—during the day for these patients (Lim, 2014). After discussion and support from the nursing staff, you develop a proposal for leadership to make 'nap time' available for all units. After collaborating with multiple departments, you are pleased to see the results of your advocacy succeed, with results of more rested patients and the additional benefit of better patient satisfaction scores (Centers for Medicare and Medicaid Services, 2013b).

When you are advocating for patients, unplanned changes do not always allow time for research and scheduling. Let's say you are covering your division this weekend. Mr. W. is a 30-year-old who is terminally ill with pancreatic cancer. He and his fiancée planned their wedding for next month, but he may not live that long. You are paged that they would like to marry this weekend if possible. You meet with the couple and talk with his nurse about the patient's ability to tolerate the ceremony and the best location. Then, you contact Legal about obtaining the license, Social Work about arrangements, Chaplaincy about the service, Dietary about the reception, the Gift Shop about flowers, and the Administrator on Call about this unplanned change. Your advocacy for Mr. (and Mrs.) W. succeeds. By the end of the weekend, the newlyweds are "honeymooning" in his room while multiple departments are basking in the afterglow, including the Administrator on Call and you!

Nurse Advocacy

In this week's staff meeting, nurses expressed concern about obtaining timely lab draws for pediatric patients with Type 1 diabetes. The phlebotomists do their best, but are needed on multiple units. The unit nurses would like to perform these draws themselves to ensure timeliness and patient safety. You and a staff RN meet with the Laboratory Director to determine the feasibility of nurse collecting lab draws for these patients. You advocate for education for the nurses by Laboratory staff to validate competency and for a pilot project to be evaluated by both the Laboratory and nursing staff (Lee-Lewandrowski & Lewandrowski, 2002). Then, you ensure adequate staffing to support the time spent by the nurses in this new procedure. After the six-week trial, you and the Laboratory Director review the evaluations as well as feedback from parents. Based on positive feedback from everyone involved and the timeliness of obtaining these lab results, the change becomes part of the standard of care on the unit.

Role of Nursing

Your advocacy extends to the role of nursing in the facility. As a nurse manager, you will serve on committees, task forces, and project teams. Your advocacy in these groups needs to reflect the standard of care. Healthcare organizations are striving to reduce CAUTI and you are invited to join your facility's CAUTI Prevention Task Force (Centers for Medicare and Medicaid Services, 2013b). After reviewing the organization's data and researching best practices, a protocol is developed and education planned. You realize that the protocol should be nurse-driven, enabling nurses to initiate catheter removal for patients who meet the criteria. At your facility, this has not been the standard of care. Your advocacy, in this case, extends to the role of nursing, and you elicit support from standards and guidelines from professional organizations as well as organizational leaders. Your diligence and advocacy pays off in a nurse-driven protocol and reduced CAUTI rates (Centers for Medicare and Medicaid Services, 2013b).

Your advocacy challenges mirror those faced by Florence in many ways. For both of you, they encompass advocacy for patients, staff, and the role of nursing.

The Importance of Communication for Nurse Leaders

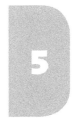

Avenues for communication have evolved since Florence's time, but the importance of communication for nurse leaders has not changed. Connecting with others is vital for better patient care and nursing practice.

Florence's Role

Written Communication

Florence Nightingale was a voracious reader with a gift for literary expression. She wrote letters constantly throughout her life and was an inveterate note-taker (Cook, 1913a). She wrote memos to herself and considered writing "a supplement for living" (Cook, 1913a, p. 93). During her life, she wrote numerous publications about health, sanitation, efficiency, hospital administration, and nursing (Cook, 1913a). Some of these publications were written by Florence, but attributed to various commissions (Cook, 1913a; Cook, 1913b). Her concern was attaining results, not on achieving credit for her work. Her *Notes Affecting the Health, Efficiency, and Hospital Administration of the British Army* and *Subsidiary Notes on the Introduction of Female Nursing into Military Hospitals in Peace and War* were self-published for presentation to influential people (Cook, 1913a). Her personal interviews and correspondence about sanitary improvement in India were noted by Indian officials. She served as a confidential advisor to the Sanitary Department at the India Office (Cook, 1913a). The volume of Florence's written work was impressive and enabled her to change health care in her time (Cook, 1913b).

Verbal Communication

Florence approached verbal communication calmly and quietly. She was assertive when necessary, but always considerate of others' feelings. In difficult interactions with some of the surgeons in the Crimea, Florence stayed calm, self-possessed, and spoke quietly. Her position in society and influential friends did not cause Florence to be overbearing. She was tactful, diplomatic, and emphasized clarity in communication (Cook, 1913a). She was aware of her influence on Ministers, the Court, and soldiers and was careful to communicate with the soldiers, always having their interest in mind. Although popular with the Crown, Florence only saw Queens and Princesses if they took a personal and practical interest in hospitals or nursing. Meetings had to be one-on-one and focused on details (Cook, 1913b). As Florence aged, she met with few people, but she always interacted with students from the Nightingale Training School and Lady Superintendents, many of whom were her protégées (Cook, 1913a). Florence's advice was widely sought and she never gave it lightly. Her emphasis on statistics carried over into her verbal communications. She valued clarity and logic and focused on action, but she was also diplomatic, sympathetic, and affectionate toward others (Cook, 1913b). Her personal touch was also valued. As she aged, Florence preferred to see one person at a time on a set schedule. She preferred her guests to talk while she listened carefully to their comments. Her active listening ability drew her visitors out and enabled her to advise and influence others in verbal communications (Cook, 1913b).

The Nurse Manager's Role

You can access multiple avenues of communication in your daily work. While Florence used verbal, written, and face-to-face communication, you are inundated with multiple electronic sources. It is easy to spend a lot of time sending and responding to email. As a new nurse manager, some attention to email is necessary, but skills in verbal, face-to-face, and written communication are as important today as they were for Florence. She knew that connecting with people resulted in better patient care, and that is an important lesson for you to learn in your new role (American Nurses Association, 2009).

Electronic Communication

Electronic communication may be a blessing or a curse for new nurse managers. You can communicate in real time with colleagues across the country and locate best practice resources. You can also spend hours checking, reading, and responding to (or deleting) emails. Email is a source of information—some important, some not. You need to develop a system that you can control for using email. You need to set limits (Rennecker & Derks, 2013). Plan a specific amount of time for this task and delete any non-essential emails so you don't end up re-reading them. Focus on actionable emails first, but be careful when responding. Many people send quick responses without proofing them. That is a recipe for disaster. Remember to read your responses carefully before you hit "send" to ensure that your reader(s) will clearly understand your meaning. There have been times when a poorly proofed email had the opposite result of what was intended. It is a good practice to save a draft response and come back later to review the content prior to sending it. When you review your draft response, look at the email as your recipient will see it initially. If there is any doubt about how your email will be received, do not send it. Opt for a face-to-face communication instead. One last piece of advice: never write or send an email when you are angry or upset. The risk is not worth using this form of communication.

Written Communication

As a new manager, you need to understand and utilize the power of the written word as Florence did. You will have many opportunities to demonstrate your skills in written communication, including policy/procedure development, proposals, business plans, project development, articles for internal publication, and even journal submissions to promote best practices. Florence honed her literary skills over a lifetime and many of her little-known publications changed peoples' lives throughout the world (Selanders & Crane, 2012; Cook, 1913a). You will communicate in writing with all levels of your organization as well as with members of other disciplines and community members. Your written communication must be clear, concise, and easy to understand. It also needs to be unbiased and complete. Remember to always check your written communication before sending forward. Spell Check is a good tool, but it is no substitute for carefully reviewing your material. Poorly chosen words may come back to haunt you because written communications have a life of their own after they leave your word processor. If you are not sure of your current writing ability, take a continuing education course at your local college or attend a community class. In this case, practice will not achieve total perfection, but your written communication skills will advance as you use them. Remember, they are essential to your success in your new role.

Verbal Communication

You engage in verbal communication throughout your day in the workplace. Some verbal communication is brief and relaxed. Other verbal exchanges may be emotionally charged for you and others. You need regular face-to-face contact with patients, family members, and staff members on your unit so you know what is happening and can address issues before they become problems (American Nurses Association, 2009). As you connect with others for better patient care, you must remember that communication is a two-way street. You will never have all the answers. No one does, but input from others is essential to your success in verbal communication. Verbal communication is a skill that you will use with all levels of your organization on a daily basis. It is important in face-to-face interactions to verify your meaning to others. Never guess how your words are being received. Ask questions, seek clarification, and rephrase responses to ensure clear understanding. In these interactions, take a lesson from Florence and practice active listening skills. No one is born with this ability, but you can develop it. Focus on the individual(s) in the conversation and really hear what is being said. Many of us love to talk and give advice. That advice will not be well received if we do not pay attention to others' response. You like to be clearly understood and you need to afford the same courtesy to others. Active listening is a skill that requires practice. Focus on not dominating the conversation. You need to really hear what the other person is trying to tell you. The benefits for both of you will be enormous. In the words of the Greek philosopher Epictetus: "We have two ears and one mouth so that we can listen twice as much as we speak" (Dictionary.com, n.d).

Remember, the more you practice active listening skills, the more effective you will be in your new role and in life.

The Importance of Career Development

6

Florence's Role

Nursing Education

As we have seen, Florence Nightingale faced adversity and obstacles in developing her career as a trained nurse (Cook, 1913b). Much of her early education resulted from home schooling in the arts and sciences. She was a diligent student who worked hard to complete assignments (Cook, 1913a). For Florence, that level of education was not sufficient for her to achieve her goal as a nurse. She didn't like religious orders in themselves, but was interested in the Institution for Deaconesses at Kaiserwerth, Germany, founded by Pastor Theodor Fliedner (Cook, 1913a). This reputable Protestant institution and nursing school on the Rhine enabled gentlewomen to serve an apprenticeship for nursing that would equip them to practice elsewhere and assume larger responsibilities (Cook, 1913a). When Florence received one of Pastor Fliedner's Annual Reports, she realized that Kaiserwerth was the sort of institution that her mother might not object to her attending (Cook, 1913a). She began this pursuit in 1846 and realized her dream in 1851 when she spent three months at Kaiserwerth. During her waiting period, Florence pursued studies on medical and sanitary subjects to prepare herself for training as a nurse (Cook, 1913a). Kaiserwerth trained volunteer nurses as deaconesses who worked in France, Switzerland, and America (Cook, 1913a). These women were Lutheran, Methodist, and Episcopalian, who were consecrated as deaconesses and received blessing in church, but took no vows (Cook, 1913a). The facility consisted of a 100-bed hospital, penitentiary with twelve inmates, an orphan asylum, and a normal school for schoolmistresses (Cook, 1913a). During Florence's stay, there were 116 deaconesses at Kaiserwerth. Ninety-four were consecrated and the rest were on probation (students) (Cook, 1913a). Everything was clean and well-ordered and training was practical, with emphasis on practice and principles (Cook, 1913a). Florence enjoyed Dr. Fliedner's lectures and the opportunity to develop her skills (Cook, 1913a). After finishing her term at Kaiserwerth, Florence returned home. Her next educational opportunity occurred in 1852, when she studied with the Catholic Sisters of Charity in Paris (Cook, 1913a). Twenty sisters managed their house and cared for nearly 200 orphans and patients at an attached hospital for aged and sick women (Cook, 1913a). Florence also went to two hospitals, a general and children's hospital, within ten minutes' walk (Cook, 1913a). She studied numerous Paris hospitals during her stay and wrote reports, statistics, and pamphlets about hospital organization and nursing arrangements in France and Germany (Cook, 1913a). She resumed her Paris studies at Maison de la Providence from June 8–July 13, 1852 (Cook, 1913a). This was the extent of her formal nursing education, but Florence didn't stop there.

Ongoing Professional Development

Florence was a lifelong student. Her interests were varied and she sought experts and mentors to increase her own knowledge. She studied sanitation with Dr. John Sutherland, a recognized expert sanitarian, and became an expert herself on the principles of sanitation (12). Her expertise translated into efforts with multiple experts to improve the health of the population (Cook, 1913a). Florence devoted significant study to the health of the Army and the Indian people (Cook, 1913b). She used her knowledge to improve the medical administration of the Army (Cook, 1913a), and became the recognized expert for sanitary progress in India (Cook, 1913b). Her study of mortality in lying-in (maternity) wards changed the function of these wards by her emphasis on cleanliness and isolation. She developed plans for sanitary lying-in (maternity) hospitals (Cook, 1913b).

Florence used her ongoing professional development in practice as seen by the examples above. Knowledge was an opportunity for her to improve the life of others and she used her knowledge in practical ways by setting high goals for herself. She mentored nursing students and Lady Superintendents to help them succeed (Cook, 1913a). Florence role-modeled the value of learning and education throughout her life and her insistence on trained nurses changed the image of nursing for the future, replacing untrained, poor quality nurses with women of character, intelligence, and skills (Cook, 1913b).

The Nurse Manager's Role

Nursing Education

There are still different avenues to attain nursing degrees. As a new nurse manager, you may have a BSN or be completing that degree. Some of you have an MSN or plan to pursue that degree. You know that formal education is important for success. Plan to meet with your supervisor/director to discuss how to include formal education in your new role. The skills and knowledge you obtain will make you a better nurse manager and the support of your leader is essential for success. Remember, Florence struggled to obtain her nursing education, and she did it a little at a time in different schools and countries (Cook, 1913a; Cook, 1913b). Your challenges are different, but real. You have multiple opportunities today to obtain further formal education. Nurses continuing their education can attend accredited institutions that offer multiple opportunities—web-based learning, study groups, self-study, and online classes. Lectures are still available, but less desirable for many nurses. Studies that can be completed on your own time demonstrate the flexibility that many nurse managers need. When you are pursuing your educational journey, remember to do what Florence did and translate your new knowledge into your practice.

Ongoing Professional Development

You also know that you have a lot to learn in your new role. Ongoing professional development must be part of your professional goals. Of course, you will attend formal leadership orientation classes, but they are only the beginning. Florence sought out experts to learn from and you need to do the same. Your organization may assign a leadership preceptor to help you learn and practice skills in budgeting, planning, monitoring, and evaluating (Cook, 1913a). You also need to seek an expert mentor as Florence did for a long-term relationship to help you increase your knowledge and expertise. This mentor may be someone from another department who can broaden your knowledge base (Ives Erickson, Jones, & Ditomassi, 2013). Of course, you will attend conferences and seminars as part of your new role. Remember, that you must translate your knowledge into practice, as Florence did. You are in a pivotal role that can improve patient care. The more learning experiences you obtain, the more effective you will be in improving others' lives. Do not forget to learn from your staff and other managers (peers). They have invaluable advice to share with you. Your professional skill development must be ongoing as Florence's was.

Reading literature is a positive step, but it is only a step. You need to constantly learn and grow in the context of your position and throughout your life. Also remember to become involved in professional nursing organizations, such as the American Nurses Association and specialty nursing organizations, to further your ongoing professional development. Their standards and practice frameworks will be excellent resources for your professional growth, and the opportunity to engage in dialogue with local and national nursing experts will be invaluable in your ongoing skill development (American Nurses Association, 2009). At this time, the Code of Ethics for Nurses is being revised, but the current edition summarizes the case for professional growth succinctly: "Continual professional growth, particularly in knowledge and skill, requires a commitment to lifelong learning. Such learning includes, but is not limited to, continuing education, networking with professional colleagues, self-study, professional reading, certification, and seeking advanced degrees. Nurses are required to have knowledge relevant to the current scope and standards of nursing practice, changing issues, concerns, controversies, and ethics," (American Nurses Association, 2001, p. 18). You, your patients, your staff, and your organization will benefit as nursing and people from all over the world benefitted from Florence's lifelong love of learning.

Developing Others

Florence's Role

Developing Nurses

When Florence arrived in the Crimea, she faced challenges managing the nurses under her command. She brought 38 nurses of her own selection (ten Catholic sisters, eight Anglican sisters, six nurses from St. John's House, and fourteen other nurses from various English hospitals), but found it difficult to find quality nurses (Cook, 1913a). Florence sent one nurse back to England at once and dismissed two or three more for poor conduct. Four of the nurses from St. John's House were unable to accept the required discipline and the hardship in the war zone and went home (Cook, 1913a). Florence made unpopular decisions to meet patient needs. She transferred her best nurses to other hospitals at times because she knew they would provide quality patient care. At these times, Florence kept less trustworthy nurses under her own direction (Cook, 1913a). Of the 38 nurses who reported to Florence, she considered 16 efficient and 5 to 6 excellent (Cook, 1913a). By the end of the war, Florence had 125 nurses under her command and her concern for their welfare was evident. She even personally cared for one of the nuns who came with her through a dangerous attack of fever (Cook, 1913a). Florence also sent a letter to Dr. Bowman, the ophthalmic surgeon, from Harley Street, and commended two of her nurses, Mrs. Roberts and Mrs. Drake, for their excellence (Cook, 1913a).

Her concern extended to the families of her nurses and she requested her sister, Lady Verney, look after the children of one of the nurses (Cook, 1913a).

While Florence was still in the Crimea, public support for her at home resulted in the establishment of the Nightingale Fund in her honor to establish a training school for nurses in England similar to Kaiserwerth (Cook, 1913a). When she returned home, Florence turned her focus to developing nursing as a profession. The Nightingale Fund was used to establish the Nightingale Training School for Nurses at St. Thomas' Hospital. It also provided Midwife training at King's College Hospital for six years (Cook, 1913a). Florence's influence on the personal and professional development of nurses at the Nightingale Training School was enormous, particularly in her later years. She regularly met with the Sisters about students' progress, conferred with medical instructors, reviewed the students' work, and became personally acquainted with many of the students there (Cook, 1913b). Florence also received regular visits from matrons, sisters, nurses, and students seeking her advice and she encouraged them to focus on education, quality patient care, and individual improvement (Cook, 1913b). Florence's influence was exemplified in the nurses she mentored—women of high character, intelligence, tact, diplomacy, and skill (12). She realized that the key to success was developing others and thus sought opportunities for them to excel. She was interested in finding superior nurses and guiding them to positions where they could demonstrate excellence. Florence was an excellent judge of character and this helped her evaluate nurses for positions in numerous facilities. She also maintained constant communication with her protégées as they assumed new roles and responsibilities. They confided in her, modeled her behavior, and sought her advice and encouragement in difficult situations. "Nightingale Nurses" from around the world benefitted from Florence's mentoring and coaching as they assumed leadership positions. One of these women was Linda Richards, America's first trained nurse, who completed her post-graduate work at the Nightingale School (Cook, 1913b). Florence also recognized the importance of promoting the excellence of these nurse leaders by commending them and their achievements to organizations and civic leaders (Cook, 1913b). Florence's pride in her mentees was reflected in their success achieved in their areas of practice. Nightingale Nurses worked as midwives, reformers of workhouse nursing, hospital nurses, and lady superintendents (Cook, 1913b). Florence's mentees were recognized for their achievements, and Florence continued to support and develop each individual as opportunities for them to excel occurred. For example, Agnes Jones was hired at Florence's request as Lady Superintendent of the Workhouse Infirmary of Liverpool to institute nursing reforms. Ms. Jones was young and intensely devoted to her work. She was educated at St.

Thomas' Hospital and Kaiserwerth. Ms. Jones met Florence in 1862 and her mentor advised her to complete her apprenticeship by completing a year of training at St. Thomas' Hospital. After that time, she began work as a nurse at the Great Northern Hospital. After an interview with Florence, she accepted the position at Liverpool to reform workhouse nursing. Ms. Jones led 12 other Nightingale Nurses to the Infirmary in collaboration with Mr. William Rathbone, a philanthropist who consulted Florence about developing a system of district (community) nursing in Liverpool. The Liverpool Infirmary was a culture shock to a refined young woman who had only been in well-run hospitals. Florence wrote Ms. Jones to strengthen her resolve in facing the appalling degradation of the male pauper (indigent) wards. She had to dismiss 35 "pauper nurses" in the first few months for drunkenness. The standard of cleanliness was poor and Florence kept communicating with her to offer advice and encouragement. Florence also mediated issues between Ms. Jones and the governor of the Infirmary. Ms. Jones consulted with Florence regularly and developed "the Nightingale touch" to get her way without upsetting the officials, much as Florence did at Harley Street. Soon, doctors asked Ms. Jones if she could take charge of the female wards too. The experiment became a success and a springboard for other reforms (Cook, 1913a). Agnes Jones is only one of many mentees of Florence Nightingale who sought opportunities for excellence after she developed their skills. Florence's support and encouragement made all the difference in their success.

Developing Support Staff

Florence learned the importance of orderlies during her work in Crimean military hospitals, where orderlies played a significant role in patient care. Florence quickly realized that she would have to influence the orderlies to affect reforms in sanitation for soldiers in the wards (Cook, 1913a). She also knew that development of these staff members was essential for quality patient care. In her words, "[t]he instruction of the Orderlies in their business was one of the main uses of us in the War hospitals" (Cook, 1913a, p. 219). She spent time with them and role-modeled nursing care for them. Her calm, gentle approach won their trust and enhanced their skills in caring for patients. She continued to press for training of orderlies after her return and succeeded when a Committee to reorganize the Army Hospital Corps in 1860 formed a corps of orderlies who were carefully selected, specially trained, and attached to regimental hospitals (Cook, 1913a). She believed that the most important function of the nurse was to educate the orderly and served as a role model for nurses in performing this function to improve patient care (Cook, 1913b).

The Nurse Manager's Role

The first point you must remember as you begin developing others is to lead by example as Florence did. Teaching, coaching, and mentoring are skills that you will use daily as you interact with staff members on your unit (Sasser, 2010). You need to know your staff and their abilities, knowledge, goals, and challenges. The support of a trusted mentor will help you succeed as a new manager. You are also responsible for developing others, both nurses and support team members. They will look to you for leadership and professional advice. Numerous education and learning opportunities exist. It is important that you guide others to appropriate resources and focus on their continued skill development. As Florence developed Agnes Jones, you will have the opportunity to develop others. She supported Agnes in a difficult new role and recognized her efforts to others. You must recognize staff for excellence, both within the unit and within the facility. Your encouragement will increase their motivation to succeed. Helping them to set and achieve goals is a significant role for you as the nurse manager.

Developing Nurses

Your nurses are individuals with varying experience and skills. As you observe their daily activities, you need to ensure that they are clinically competent. Competence is a requisite for autonomy and control over practice (American Academy of Nursing, 2010). As Florence evaluated her nurses in the Crimea, you will evaluate the skills of your nurses to determine your stellar performers, average performers, and those who are not meeting care delivery standards. You cannot just focus on your best performers. Development is a priority for all nurses on the unit as illustrated by the following three *Values in Action!* scenarios.

Values in Action!

Tara

Tara, a recent graduate, has been on your unit for eight months. This is her first nursing position and she is well liked by staff and patients. Tara is very social and enjoys interacting with others. However, she has made two medication errors in the past six weeks. One resulted in an omission of a scheduled antibiotic. The other resulted in administration of the wrong dose of a Beta Blocker when Tara didn't note the change in dosage on the physician's order. You have counseled Tara after each incident and today you want to observe her 0900 medication administration. The unit has a separate medication room for privacy in medication preparation. Tara leaves the door open so she can see what is happening on the unit as she prepares her 0900 meds. You observe the entire med pass. Tara does well with patient identification, medication administration, and documentation. Afterward you talk with her about your observations. Tara's need for social contact affects the necessity to focus on the task at hand when preparing medications. You cannot tolerate inattention to this vital aspect of patient care and Tara's performance must meet acceptable standards starting now. After counseling and teaching Tara, you develop an action plan with her input to improve her performance with medication administration—an action plan with defined objectives, specific action steps, timelines, and accountability. You also plan for review, monitoring, and designated meetings with Tara to ensure compliance with the action plan and acceptable performance with medication administration (Association for Nursing Professional Development, 2013).

Values in Action!

Melody

Melody is an experienced nurse and has worked on your unit for five years. She is a competent employee who always completes her work in a timely and capable manner. She attends unit meetings, but doesn't volunteer for committees or task forces. Melody's main focus is her family and her job is a way to provide extra income for her children's needs. Melody is a reliable nurse who provides good patient care. You would like to develop Melody professionally, but are unsure how to go about it. Then, one day Melody comes to your office about one of her assigned patients. The patient, a young woman with abdominal pain, is very anxious, particularly when her husband visits. Melody talked with her as she changed her IV and recognized signs of emotional abuse—e.g. depression, fearfulness, meekness when husband was present (Hamel, 2014). Melody is very concerned about her patient's welfare, but the woman was admitted yesterday and no one has mentioned any concern until now. You ask Melody how she is so sure about the abuse. She hesitates a moment and replies, "My mother was abused and I work with local abuse victims in my role as a parish nurse." Needless to say, you had no idea about this. You contact social work and initiate a report. After thorough investigation, the patient confirms Melody's suspicions and is directed to a local social agency for support. You commend Melody for her diligence and critical assessment skills. You also coach her to teach other nurses how to recognize signs and symptoms of abuse beyond physical appearance. Of course, she doesn't want to take time from her family, but she will do a video demonstration that can be shared with other units as well. After the video is distributed and other hospital staff members realize Melody's dedication to eliminating abuse, her expertise in the topic makes her a valued resource for other units (on on-duty time) and other parish nurses in the community. Melody is a competent nurse with a passion. You have found that passion and cultivated it for the benefit of future patients and community members as well as Melody herself.

Values in Action!

Mike

Mike is a superstar on your unit. He is the first to volunteer, whether it is for a committee, task force, or council. He conducts unit audits and serves as a charge nurse and preceptor. Mike is a joy to work with and serves as an informal leader for his colleagues. You may think that because he is doing so well, you don't have to be concerned about his development. You would be wrong. Florence believed that nursing is a progressive art and to stand still is to go backward (Cook, 1913b). As she developed superior nurses for advanced roles, you owe it to Mike to mentor him as he defines his future goals and aspirations. As you listen to Mike, he confides that he loves teaching as both charge nurse and preceptor. He would enjoy a position in staff development and one is coming open soon. However, he is unsure about presenting to large groups, particularly at orientation. That is a skill he has not experienced in his clinical practice. With his permission, you contact the manager of staff development and arrange for Mike to present a specific skill at the next orientation. Then, you ensure that he has time to prepare his presentation and that his patients are covered (if you have to do it yourself) while he is at the orientation. The plan is a success! Mike enjoyed talking with the large group and participant evaluations were positive. You know that when Mike applies for the staff development position, he will be successful. Although, you hate to lose his skills on your unit, you have contributed to his future success by giving him the opportunity to develop a new skill set. A key aspect in your role as nurse manager includes teaching, coaching, and mentoring nurses like Mike.

Developing Support Staff

Florence was concerned about developing orderlies, and you should feel the same about your patient care technicians. Another goal of yours should be to help support staff members succeed. Some of these individuals may be interested in a nursing career. Others may want a career in another aspect of health care. Still, others may be satisfied in their current role. How you develop your support team members through mentoring, educating, and coaching is illustrated in the following *Values in Action!* scenarios.

Values in Action!

Mandy

Mandy is a patient care assistant (PCA) who has been employed on your unit for several years. She is in her 40s and is a respected team member. She provides competent patient care and promptly reports abnormal findings to the patient's nurse. Mandy enjoys patient care and seems satisfied with her job. You are rounding on the unit and decide to help Mandy change a bed while the patient is in the shower. It will give you a chance to talk with her. As you work together, you ask her where she sees herself in two years. She seems startled by the question and replies, "probably here." You persist and ask her about her future goals. She says she enjoys working with patients and staff members and performing physical care. She likes making patients feel and look good. Suddenly, you have an idea for Mandy's development through education. The Division's clinical nurse specialist (CNS) is working on an initiative to prevent non-ventilator hospital-acquired pneumonia for the older population on your unit. One of the interventions is improved oral care and new oral care equipment (Quinn et al., 2014). You talk with Mandy about this initiative and she is excited about being part of the process. You connect the CNS and Mandy, and she becomes the unit champion for the new oral protocol to improve patients' oral health. She is now the resident unit expert on oral care and continues to enjoy her PCA role.

Values in Action!

Jeff

Jeff is a new PCA on the unit, but he is rapidly making himself indispensable to the nurses and patients. He is eager and enthusiastic about learning and is the best hire you and the staff members of the unit interview team have made in a long time. You meet with Jeff to recognize how well he is doing and to see how you can help him meet his goals. He is in his late 20s and was a medic in the Army before being hired on the unit. Jeff wants to become a registered nurse and can enroll under the GI Bill. However, he also needs to earn a living. Jeff has checked local schools, but flexibility is limited so he is at a standstill. You mentor Jeff by introducing him to accredited distance-learning nursing programs. You both investigate several of these programs, and Jeff is able to find one that meets his needs and permits him to work while going to school. You also help him adjust his schedule as needed for on-campus requirements (Andrews, 2014). Flash forward a couple of years. Jeff is now an RN and ready to meet with your interview team. You will have to hire a new PCA, but the unit has gained a dedicated RN. That's a win-win!

Values in Action!

Molly

Molly is a PCA who has been employed on the unit for 11 months. She is in her early 20s and gives adequate patient care. She often "forgets" to keep the patient's nurse informed of changes in condition. Yesterday, a diabetic patient displayed symptoms of hypoglycemia and Molly didn't report this until the nurse found the patient going into shock. Today, you are meeting with Molly to discuss the situation and develop an action plan to improve Molly's job performance. During the conversation, Molly mentions that the PCA role is not what she really wants to do. She is taking business courses to become an administrative assistant. You ask if she has explored positions closer to her goal and she says she looks regularly, but is not qualified for open administrative assistant positions until she completes her education. Since Molly is not well-suited for patient care and patients are not benefitting from her presence, you begin coaching her for future professional development as you develop the action plan. Molly is qualified for receptionist positions within the organization based on those job descriptions. This role would be an opportunity for her to practice skills that she will use later in the administrative assistant role. Within two months, Molly is transferred to a receptionist position in the organization. Until her transfer, Molly continues to meet the steps in her action plan by promptly reporting any changes in a patient's condition to the nurse. Your coaching has benefitted Molly's future career path and, most of all, your patients.

Where Do You Go From Here?

Development of your team is essential to ensure the delivery of quality patient care and that must be your ultimate goal. Give team members the opportunity to excel and reward them for achieving that excellence. Your success is reflected in the success of your team and their achievements. Florence understood that helping others develop their skills and succeed would benefit reforms in patient care. You have the same opportunity in your new role and that is exciting. Someday, you will have your own story about how you helped a nurse or support staff member seek and find opportunities to excel. Florence's legacy was the development of professional nursing and her teaching, coaching, and mentoring was essential to that legacy. You will have many opportunities to create your own legacy during your career; teaching, coaching, and mentoring others to achieve their goals will be essential to your legacy as a nurse leader.

Community Partnerships

8

Florence's Role

Improving the Health of the Community

Florence Nightingale's community was the world and she spent most of her life improving the health of her community (Cook, 1913a; Cook, 1913b). In her role as Lady Superintendent at Harley Street, Florence facilitated transfers of patients to convalescent homes to ensure follow-up care in the community (Cook, 1913a). Her personal concern for soldiers during her service in the Crimea resulted in the establishment of a reading room and classrooms for them (Cook, 1913a). Her leadership continued after her return to England, where she led the movement to increase these facilities to help soldiers attain useful employment (Cook, 1913b). Florence's concern for sanitation reforms permeated many of the community causes she supported over the years (Cook, 1913a; Cook, 1913b). While at Embley with her sick mother in 1866, Florence worked on the health of citizens in Romsey and Winchester by focusing on drains to reduce local mortality (Cook, 1913b). Her expertise in sanitary science was influential on communities from England to India and even the United States (Cook, 1913b). Florence's interest in sanitation continued in her later years and became an impetus for the district nursing movement. In 1890, she spent time at Claydon, her country home, and became interested in nurses as health missioners (officials). The district health officer trained these nurses by presenting classes and lectures as well as taking them with him on visits. Then, they completed an independent examination. Those who passed the test completed a probationary practicum and received certificates as health missioners (Cook, 1913b). Florence enlisted recruits, focused on simple sanitary instruction, considered syllabi and exam papers, corresponded with other technical education committees, and wrote memos and letters on the subject of sanitation, including a paper on rural hygiene (Cook, 1913b).

Community Service
Florence personally performed community service from her youth, when she visited the poor in her local community with her mother (Cook, 1913a). During a winter in Rome (1847–1848), Florence found a poor girl on the street and paid for her care and education at the orphanage of Dames Du Sacre Coeur for many years (Cook, 1913a). After her return from the Crimea, Florence spent time with her mother at Lea Hurst and devoted herself to her poorer neighbors in the area. She helped establish a village coffee house and a village library as well as organizing mothers' meetings. She served as a promoter for the National Health Insurance Scheme (Plan) for the neighborhood by employing a doctor to care for the ill and infirmed at her own expense. She also commissioned the village school teacher to give extra tuition to promising students (Cook, 1913b).

The Nurse Manager's Role
Improving the Health of the Community
As a nurse manager, you will have opportunities to improve the health of your community. Florence devoted significant energy to improving community sanitation throughout the world, a cause that was her passion (Cook, 1913b). You need to find your own passion. Your clinical unit may help determine the causes you promote. If you manage a neonatal intensive-care unit (NICU), the March of Dimes Foundation may be an organization you support because of the services it provides to NICU graduates. If you manage an oncology unit, the American Cancer Society's local chapter may elicit your support because of the services it provides for your patients. Your organization will also support numerous local non-profits and can provide you an opportunity to get involved in improving the health of your community. It is not necessary to join every charitable activity. Select those that you believe in and get involved! Florence was never a passive participant in community health activities. She was a leader, and this is your opportunity to develop your leadership skills while making your community healthier. It is important not to narrowly focus on your daily activities. This is a chance to meet people, network, develop positive

relationships, collaborate with other leaders, and truly make a positive difference where you live.

Community Service

Florence's community service was not all nursing-related. She gave of her time and resources to help those in need. The hospital is not your only world as a nurse manager. You have numerous opportunities to be visible and involved in direct community service. Consider the possibility of spending time helping in a local food back or soup kitchen, or even helping grade school children improve their reading readiness skills. If you wish to serve community residents by using your nursing and leadership skills, consider presenting health programs at local schools or senior centers. You probably have numerous ideas of your own by now. Select the ones that will meet your personal desires and the needs of your community members. You will get as much pleasure as Florence did in serving your community.

Modeling Excellence in Care Delivery

Florence's Role
Professional Practice Framework

Florence established the first theoretical foundation for nursing (conceptual framework) in her *Notes on Nursing* (American Nurses Credentialing Center, 2008), when she described the nurse's role in maintaining balance between the patient (client) and the environment to prevent the patient from expending unnecessary energy that would impede "[t]he reparative process which Nature has instituted" (Nightingale, 1992, p. 5). She based her environmental theory on four assumptions (Nightingale, 1992):

1. Five elements are essential for healthful houses: "pure air, pure water, efficient drainage, cleanliness, and light" (p. 14).

2. A healthy environment is essential to healing. Nurses must "...put the patient in the best condition for nature to act upon him" (p. 75).

3. Nurses must accurately observe the patient and "...what symptoms indicate improvement—what the reverse—which are of importance—which are of none—which are the evidence of neglect—and of what kind of neglect" (p. 59). Nurses must then precisely report on the patient's status to the physician.

4. Nursing is an art. Nurses have their own role in patients' journeys to health by supporting the medical plan, but not being subservient because "nature alone cures" (p. 74).

Florence's major concepts encompassed nursing, the environment and its impact on patients, and health promotion (Nightingale, 1992). When a patient experiences stress due to environmental factors, nursing observations must note the patient's reaction to the stressor. Then, the nurse must take appropriate interventions to reduce the stressor and give the patient an opportunity to heal (Nightingale, 1992). Florence also applied her professional practice model when caring for healthy, as well as sick individuals (Nightingale, 1992, pg. 23). Today, Florence's professional practice framework is considered a middle range theory because of its concern with specific experiences, appropriateness for empirical testing, and potential to guide nursing practice (Peterson & Bredow, 2009). Although Florence's environmental theory would require further development to address today's environmental challenges, it serves as a dynamic beginning for the progression of the nursing profession and a template for future nurses—and theorists.

Care Delivery Structure

Florence also defined her care delivery structure in her *Notes on Nursing* when she specified how nurses should implement her environmental theory in their clinical practice. Florence believed that the nurse's goal is to help the patient stay in balance with their environment. The nurse could do this by adjusting the environment to counteract the patient's response to their surroundings (Nightingale, 1992). Florence's plan of care included attention to physical stressors that impeded nature's ability to cure the patient (Nightingale, 1992). These stressors include lack of ventilation, chilling, lack of light, noise, lack of variety (in color and activities to relieve boredom), lack of bedding changes, lack of personal cleanliness, poor nutrition, and false cheerfulness (Nightingale, 1992). Florence left specific instructions for nurses in delivering care on a daily basis. The nurse had the following responsibilities and accountabilities:

1. The first rule of nursing: "[K]eep the air he breathes as pure as the external air, without chilling him" (Nightingale, 1992, p. 8). Since hospital rooms did not have regular air exchanges, Florence recommended opening windows so the patient could breathe fresh air. Today, that would be unacceptable, but in 1859, it was a best practice (Nightingale, 1992).

2. Communicate with the patient: Inform him when you are leaving and when you will return (Nightingale, 1992). Florence understood that the nurse had to leave the bedside at times. She also recognized the importance of keeping patients informed while developing a sense of trust between nurse and patient. This is still applicable today in health care (Ives Erickson, Jones, & Ditomassi, 2013).

3. Manage the patient's care to ensure that his care will continue uninterrupted in your absence—ensure that everyone else performs assigned duties correctly (Nightingale, 1992). Florence understood that delegation

was necessary in patient care, but that the nurse maintained responsibility and accountability for patient care. Today's *Nursing: Scope and Standards of Practice* reflects Florence's care delivery model in care coordination and collaboration between care providers (American Nurses Association, 2010).

4. Reduce unnecessary noise levels so the patient can rest: Florence's emphasis on quiet remains applicable in today's hospitals (Nightingale, 1992; Murphy, Bernardo, & Dalton, 2013; Ives Erickson, Jones, & Ditomassi, 2013).

5. Avoid monotony and encourage variety in objects and colors to help the patient recover. Florence knew that people were positively affected by bright flowers, lights, and beautiful paintings and wall hangings (Nightingale, 1992). Today, hospitals have incorporated art throughout their facilities. Patient rooms with outside views and a variety of lighting also make the patient's stay more pleasant and assist in recovery.

6. Make mealtime a pleasant experience by timing meals based on patient needs, offering frequent nourishment, and attention to quality in the diet (Nightingale, 1992).

7. Ensure that bed linens are clean and that the patient is well-supported in bed to prevent bedsores and facilitate comfort (Nightingale, 1992). Today, we have specialty beds that Florence never dreamed of, but her advice for position changes is applicable to our nursing practice so we can reduce hospital-acquired pressure ulcers (HAPU) (Centers for Medicare and Medicaid Services, 2013a).

8. Environmental and personal cleanliness was imperative for Florence in daily patient care. Florence espoused frequent hand washing by nurses as well as providing detailed instructions about bathing patients. Today, hand hygiene is an integral factor in reducing the transmission of pathogenic microorganisms to patients and healthcare staff (Centers for Disease Control and Prevention, 2002).

9. Carefully observe and assess the patient to obtain accurate information to concisely share with the doctor "for the sake of saving life and increasing health and comfort" (Nightingale, 1992, p. 70). Florence's emphasis on closely observing and assessing the patient during daily care is as appropriate now as it was in 1859 (Ives Erickson, Jones, & Ditomassi, 2013).

Florence's care delivery structure incorporated her professional practice framework into the daily practice of nurses in the mid-nineteenth century. It is important to understand that today's nursing theories, professional practice models, and care delivery systems owe Florence Nightingale thanks for establishing the theoretical foundation of the modern nursing profession and significantly improving care delivery in her lifetime.

The Nurse Manager's Role
Professional Practice Framework

Now that you are aware of Florence's contribution to nursing and patients, you need to understand the theoretical framework and professional practice model at your facility. This is not just an intellectual exercise. It is vital that you as a nurse manager can express how the model reflects its theoretical basis because it will affect patient care on your unit. The Application Manual Magnet Recognition Program comprehensively describes a professional practice model as

...a schematic description of a system, theory, or phenomenon that depicts how nurses practice, collaborate, communicate, and develop professionally to provide the highest quality care for those served by the organization (e.g. patients, families, community). The Professional Practice Model illustrates the alignment and integration of nursing practice with the mission, vision, philosophy, and values that nursing has adapted. (American Nurses Credentialing Center, 2008, p. 28)

Let's illustrate this by examining two middle range nursing theories (conceptual frameworks) and their implications as professional practice models in a healthcare organization (American Nurses Credentialing Center, 2008).

Theory 1—Jean Watson's Theory of Human Caring

Watson's Theory of Human Caring considers caring the essence of nursing and stresses the importance of the relationship between the nurse and the client (patient). This relationship enables the client to increase his knowledge base, assume control of his care, and promote changes in his health.

Watson's Theory is based on the following Assumptions (Watson, 2012).

1. Caring:
    a. is interpersonal;
    b. involves "carative factors" resulting in satisfaction of certain human needs;
    c. promotes health and individual or family growth;
    d. accepts a person as he or she is now and as what he or she may become;
    e. can develop potential while letting the person choose his or her best action at a given point in time;
    f. is complementary to the science of curing; and
    g. is central to nursing.

2. Transpersonal caring:
    a. transcends time, space, and physical presence;
    b. signifies a spirit-to-spirit connection between nurse and patient;
    c. creates a caring field beyond the ego level of both nurse and patient;
    d. results in higher energy giving the patient more access to inner healing;
    e. is communicated by the nurse's authentic presence in a caring relationship;
    f. often uses noninvasive, nonintrusive, natural modalities; and
    g. promotes self-knowledge, self-control, and self-healing.

Example 1

If your nursing organization has adopted Jean Watson's Theory of Human Caring as the professional practice model, you must ensure that care delivery on your unit reflects these concepts. Your oncology unit's inpatient population undergoes arduous chemotherapy, radioactive implants, and surgery. Your nurses pride themselves on adhering to Oncology Nursing Society (ONS) practice standards and competencies in their daily practice (Putting Evidence into Practice, n.d.). Now they need to integrate these practice standards and their clinical expertise within the professional practice model based on Watson's work (Ives Erickson, Jones, & Ditomassi, 2013; Watson, 2012). Alan is a 64-year-old patient whose recent lobectomy results have revealed stage IV lung cancer. Alan has been estranged from his family for many years and has no significant support system. He is depressed and non-communicative and his oncologist has initiated a psychiatric referral to help Alan deal with his feelings and anxiety. His primary nurse, Abby, understands that ONS interventions to alleviate anxiety include educating the patient about symptoms, treatments, services and resources; providing care and responding to disease-related concerns; and to utilizing problem-solving strategies to help the patient cope with cancer (Putting Evidence into Practice, n.d.). You talk with Abby about how she can implement the professional practice model with ONS practice standards and competencies to develop a caring relationship with Alan. She is aware that the professional practice model requires her to be authentic and truly present in her interactions with him. In addition to implementing ONS's Putting Evidence into Practice for alleviating anxiety, Abby plans Alan's care visits to spend time with him when not physically providing care. She tells him, "I am here for you" and sits quietly at his bedside. At first, he doesn't respond, but her acceptance of Alan eventually evolves into a transpersonal caring relationship that helps Alan deal with his diagnosis and allows him to take control of his treatment plan with Abby's support (Watson, 2012). You facilitate a meeting with the other team members so Abby can share this change to Alan's care plan and enlist their support. Abby's colleagues support her interventions with Alan, so she has uninterrupted time at his bedside. She has integrated professional standards and relationship-based care to create the caring environment that Alan needs. Abby also benefits from this relationship, which enhances the quality of care she will provide for future patients. Both nurse and patient are changed forever by this experience (Watson, 2012).

Advanced transpersonal caring incorporates ethical and interpersonal caring along with planned modalities that respect comfort, healing, harmony, balance, wholeness, and well-being (Watson, 2012).

Now that you understand Jean Watson's theoretical framework for the Theory of Human Caring, the next step is to see how Watson's theory became a professional practice model for nursing in a healthcare organization. Watson's major concepts (i.e. definitions for society, human being, health, nursing, actual caring occasion, and transpersonal concept) are diagrammed and integrated with the organization's and nursing's philosophy, mission, vision, and values to create a framework for care delivery. The schematic depiction serves as a visual guide for nursing care delivery on a day-to-day basis.

Since no single nursing theory is applicable to each healthcare organization, it is important to select a theoretical framework that is meaningful to the practice setting.

Let's examine a contrasting nursing theory to illustrate this point.

Theory 2—Madeline Leininger's Theory of Transcultural Nursing

Leininger's assumptions differ from Watson's with their emphasis on cultural care and diversity. These assumptions are (Leininger & McFarland, 2002):

1. Culturally related care:
   a. is practiced differently in different cultures, but there are some common aspects about care in all cultures;
   b. is influenced by all aspects of the culture, e.g. spiritual, social, political, educational, economic, technological, historical, and environmental;
   c. is present for all cultures, but caring may have different expressions, actions, meanings, patterns, and lifestyles;
   d. includes generic or folk healthcare practices as well as cultural similarities and differences between providers and patients;
   e. is essential with caring for human survival, growth, health, well-being, healing, and ability to deal with handicaps and death; and
   f. is a central focus of nursing and may occur without cure.

2. Nursing as transcultural care:
   a. explains and predicts nursing care occurrences to guide nursing practice;
   b. has a central purpose to serve human beings and contributes to clients' well-being;

    c. is beneficial only when clients are known by the nurse who uses their patterns, expressions, and cultural values in appropriate and meaningful ways; and

    d. must be compatible with and respectful of clients' lifestyle, belief, and values to avoid client stress, noncompliance, cultural conflicts, and/or ethical or moral concerns.

Leininger's major concepts are:

- definition of transcultural nursing
- ethno nursing
- professional nursing caring
- cultural congruent nursing care
- health
- human beings
- worldview
- cultural and social structure dimensions
- environmental context
- culture
- culture care
- culture care diversity
- culture care universality

These major concepts are diagrammed and integrated with the organization's philosophy, mission, vision, and values to create a framework for care delivery. The schematic depiction serves as a visual guide for nursing care delivery on a day-to-day basis (Leininger & McFarland, 2002).

Although each theory uses 'caring' in its assumptions and major concepts, the focus is different and nursing must carefully select its own theoretical foundation and professional practice model to establish a framework for nursing practice (Ives Erickson, Jones, & Ditomassi, 2013).

Care Delivery Structure

Now that you understand how professional practice models represent nursing theories, it is time to discuss a vital aspect of the professional practice model—the care delivery model. As a manager, you want your nurses to deliver high-quality, cost-effective, and patient-centered care. As Florence used key concepts from her model to educate nurses for quality, patient-centered care, you need to examine the schematic of your professional practice model to achieve positive outcomes in nursing care delivery.

Example 2

You are the manager of the Pediatric Cardiovascular Unit at a tertiary care facility and the nursing department has just adopted Leininger's Transcultural Nursing Theory as the conceptual framework for nursing practice. Her major concepts are depicted in the professional practice model for application in nursing care delivery. Your patient population is relatively homogeneous, but that is about to change. Martha is a four-month old who was born with a congenital heart defect. She is being admitted for open-heart surgery to correct Tetralogy of Fallot—a congenital malformation described as an abnormal opening in the septum between the ventricles resulting in the misplacement of the aorta so it receives blood from both ventricles, narrowing of the pulmonary artery, and right ventricular enlargement (Dictionary. com, n.d.). Martha was born in a community hospital. She initially went home with mild cyanosis. In the past week, her cyanosis has increased and she now requires surgery. Martha's family is Amish and your unit is not familiar with this culture. You begin to research the Amish culture and health care to ensure culturally competent nursing care for this patient and family (Purnell, 2013). Their dress and mannerisms reflect a distinct culture of social isolation and religious community. You realize that seeking help from healthcare providers is accepted by the Amish culture when necessary. They are open to use of medical technology to improve their health, and their health-seeking behaviors are similar to the rest of the country. However, they feel that this requires them to go outside their own people and cross a cultural threshold as they enter a healthcare facility (Purnell, 2013). The Amish also have solid bonds with family and church. This means that multigenerational family presence will be important in Martha's care and providers need to support this. You also understand that, although the Amish speak English, many family members will converse in Deitsch or Pennsylvania German (Purnell, 2013). When providing verbal information, nurses must realize that the Amish may not know what we see as general knowledge. Verification of learning is essential to ensure the family's understanding (Purnell, 2013). You share your knowledge with your nursing team and plan for Martha's care using Leininger's concepts from your professional practice model. Martha arrives with her parents and grandparents. You and the nursing team include her extended family in Martha's care planning. Since it is important for her family members to play an active role in Martha's care, her primary nurse encourages their involvement. She also ensures that each family member is included in information sharing and that they understand the meaning of verbal communications (Leininger & McFarland, 2002). She demonstrates culturally competent care by her inclusiveness (Leininger & McFarland, 2002). The primary nurse documents these interventions in Martha's care plan and addresses them in the shift report to ensure consistency in her care delivery (Ives Erickson, Jones, & Ditomassi, 2013).)

In each of the above examples, the nurses adapted the care delivery model to the individualized needs of the patient. This is an important point to understand. Care delivery reflects the professional practice model, but must be tailored to the clinical setting. You need to examine approaches to care delivery for your specific patient population with your nursing team to ensure patient-centered care as Florence did in her *Notes on Nursing* (Nightingale, 1992, pg. 20). Your patients, families, and nurses will all benefit from this dialogue.

Resource and Fiscal Management

10

Florence's Role

Managing Material Resources

Florence's initial foray into fiscal management began at Harley Street where she successfully reduced medical expenses. This was impressive in a time when men made financial decisions (Cook, 1913a). She also ensured that material resources were put in place to increase efficiency during the building process for the new hospital. The resources included a call system, a hot water supply, and a lift (elevator) (Cook, 1913a). These material resources are routine in today's hospitals, but were innovative in 1853. Florence's management of material resources excelled during her time in the Crimea. When she arrived, the wards lacked essential provisions for care delivery including furniture, adequate sheets, surgical, and medical supplies (Cook, 1913a). The Purveyor-General (military supply officer) had contracted for washing of hospital bedding and patients' linen, but Florence discovered that they were washed in cold water and subsequently must be destroyed because they were full of vermin (Cook, 1913a). She used her private funds and funds from readers of the Times to acquire a house, have the Engineer's Office install boilers, and hire soldiers' wives to do the washing in hot water. Now that sick soldiers had clean linen, Florence turned her attention to another material resource—extra diet kitchens (Cook, 1913a). All cooking was done at one end of the huge hospital and it took

3 to 4 hours to serve a meal to all patients, whose beds extended from three to four miles in the building. One of Florence's actions was to open two extra diet kitchens in different parts of the hospital so the patients could eat more promptly. These successes led to Florence's role as Purveyor-Auxiliary to the Scutari hospitals. She did not anticipate this role in the beginning. It evolved as she assessed the patients' needs and the material resources available. Florence described this in a letter to Sidney Herbert on January 4, 1855: "I am a kind of General Dealer in socks, shirts, knives and forks, wooden spoons, tin baths, tables and forms, cabbage and carrots, operating tables, towels and soap, small tooth combs, precipitate for destroying lice, scissors, bedpans and stump pillows" (Cook, 1913a, p.200). To her credit, Florence never issued supplies until requested by the medical officers and only after asking the Purveyor if he could supply these items (Cook, 1913a). Since the Purveyor was slow and his process was unwieldy, Florence's stores supplied sick soldiers from the British, Prussian, and Turkish armies. In this role, she carefully dispensed articles after receipt of requisitions and signatures (Cook, 1913a). Based on her experiences with distribution of material resources, Florence developed a plan for the systematic organization of hospitals based on centralization of kitchens, furniture, clothing, and cleaning (Cook, 1913a).

Managing Human Resources
Florence's management of human resources began in Harley Street where her unique call system increased the efficiency and effectiveness of her nurses. Patient bells rang in the hallway outside the nurse's door on that floor, and a valve opened when the bell rang and stayed open so the nurse knew who called her. She also ensured that the nurse could remain on her assigned floor except for her meal periods (Cook, 1913a). In the Crimea, Florence's attention focused on management of the orderlies. The orderlies played a significant role in patient care, but were largely untrained. She educated them and recommended that they "be well paid, well fed, well housed" (Cook, 1913a, p.226). In 1884, Lord Wolseley, commander in the Egyptian Campaign, supported her assertion made many years before that nurses should monitor and train orderlies in military hospitals (Cook, 1913b). She extended her management of human resources by addressing the nurses and probationers of the Nightingale School at St. Thomas' Hospital. In one of these letters (May 23, 1873), she extolled "the pleasures of administration which ... means only learning to manage a Ward well" (Nightingale, 2012, p.28). In another (May 16, 1888), Florence described the nurse's calling to dedicate herself to the benefit of the patient by meeting all his needs (Nightingale, 2012). Her rigorous involvement with the students over many years groomed them as the next generation of nurse leaders (Cook, 1913b).

The Nurse Manager's Role

You must use the organization's and your department's resources effectively and efficiently when and where they are needed. This is not a chapter on finance and budgeting because you will receive that education as part of your manager orientation. This is one step beyond planning your capital budget and monitoring your unit operational and staffing budgets monthly. Managing material and human resources requires innovative and proactive tactics that Florence displayed throughout her career (Cook, 1913a; Cook, 1913b). This is your opportunity to meet Standard of Professional Performance 14 of the Nursing Administration: Scope and Standards of Practice. It reads, "[t]he nurse administrator considers factors related to safety, effectiveness, cost, and impact on practice in the planning and delivery of nursing and other services" (American Nurses Association, 2009, p.42).

Managing Material Resources

Let's see how you can meet this Standard of Professional Performance while managing your material resources. Your OB Unit has been remodeled over the years, but is still located in the older part of the facility. The main entrance normally has someone located at the desk to direct visitors and watch for any problems. There is a stairwell at the rear of the unit, which staff members use to access Central Services two floors below and the employee parking lot. One of your staff nurses, Betsy, has just returned from the Association of Women's Health, Obstetric, and Neonatal Nurses (AWHONN) Conference and is meeting with you to plan a program she will present to her colleagues about best practices in maternal–child health. As you talk, she mentions one of the display booths from XYZ Health Care about a unique new infant security system that excited her. You already have a security system in place so you wonder how unique it can be. You ask Betsy to leave the literature about the system for your review. After she departs to start her shift, you casually leaf through the handout. Then, it occurs to you that this system is truly innovative and may be just what your unit needs to thwart infant abduction. The current system uses a chip inside the infant's bracelet to trigger alarms and close doors at both entrances. However, after removing the bracelet, an abductor could simply put the infant in a large purse or bag and go down the backstairs to exit the building. XYZ's system also uses the bracelet with a chip inside, but the bracelet must be removed by placing an employee's registered thumbprint over the chip. If it is cut off without being deactivated in this manner, the alarm will sound and all doors will automatically shut and lock. It also has a battery-activated back up if power outages occur and is immune to false alarms. Since it requires registering all qualified OB staff members, the system is more expensive than your current one. You contact the representative and investigate the cost-benefit ratio for this change. The initial cost will be $25,400 with annual maintenance cost of $2,500 for a five-year period. Your present system's contract is up for renewal at the end of the year and costs $2,000/year currently. You meet with your Director and the Risk Manager to discuss increased patient safety along with the cost–benefit ratio of the XYZ system using a SWOT (strengths, weaknesses, opportunities, threats) Analysis (Association for Nursing Professional Development, 2013; Rundio & Wilson, 2010). After eliciting their support, you prepare a detailed business case (plan) for switching to the XYZ security product and present it to Senior Nursing Leadership for endorsement (Association for Nursing Professional Development, 2013). Then, it moves forward to Budgeting and Finance for addition to the capital budget. The process is time consuming, but the results are positive. Your unit will have a new material resource—the XYZ infant security system that is effective, efficient, and technologically innovative. Most important of all, it provides an added element of safety for infants and their families (American Nurses Association, 2009). Florence would certainly approve of your results.

Managing Human Resources
Using the example above, you publically recognize Betsy for bringing you the information about the XYZ security system. You wouldn't have made the change without her input. That vital aspect of managing human resources is often neglected as an opportunity to recognize and build trust (American Academy of Nursing, 2010). The nurse manager doesn't work in isolation. Your team will guide you to innovative approaches that will improve the care on the unit and in the facility if you develop and listen to them. One of your responsibilities is to ensure your nurses understand the operational and staffing budgets, particularly related to their day-to-day activities. Their input can assist you in planning for equipment and technology purchases as Betsy did with the security system. Their knowledge of staffing and scheduling can ensure delivery of patient-centered care even in busy situations with limited resources. If you support your nurses to function together as a team and maintain clinical autonomy over their nursing practice, concern for the patient will dominate their actions and yours (American Academy of Nursing, 2010). Let's look at an example to illustrate this statement.

You share the above statement about teamwork and clinical autonomy with all new hires. Then, your preceptors guide them to attain competencies and diverse clinical experiences. You collaborate with the preceptors, charge nurses, and other staff nurses to ensure that these nurses have experiences that enable them to exercise clinical judgment to anticipate and prevent negative patient outcomes as they grow into their new roles (Ives Erickson, Jones, & Ditomassi, 2013). Chad joined your CHF unit a year ago as an RN and is now performing at a competent level. He is comfortable in most clinical situations and uses resources readily to ensure his patients receive quality care. Chad has become a valued team player, and volunteers when the unit is busy. He also actively seeks new learning opportunities to enhance his nursing skills. Quality reports show an increase in readmissions within 30 days of discharge for CHF patients and you discuss this concern with the staff at unit meetings (Centers for Medicare and Medicaid Services, 2013b). Chad expresses concern about patients' knowledge of home care post-discharge and offers to investigate how this aspect relates to readmissions. You help him survey readmitted patients and he also talks with other team members about approaches to ensure patients' understanding about diet, exercise, medications, and follow-up care. Everyone agrees that the day of discharge is busy, and therefore patients don't pay attention to the huge volume of information they receive. Chad does a literature review and discovers the "teach-back method when providing discharge education" (Haney & Shepherd, 2014, p. 50). You and Chad share this information with the unit staff at unit meetings. A key group of volunteers, with Chad as leader, develops teach-back sessions for CHF patients during their hospitalizations. These sessions begin while patients are hospitalized and are reinforced as needed until discharge. At Chad's suggestion, the nurses also call the patients the day after discharge to address any questions or concerns. The next month's quality report shows significant reduction in readmission of CHF patients within 30 days after discharge. Besides recognizing Chad and his team on the unit, you arrange for them to present their innovative approach to the Quality Council, where they receive kudos for their success. As Florence groomed her probationers to become nurse leaders, you have an opportunity and obligation to groom your staff nurses for professional advancement as you meet this Standard of Professional Performance (Cook, 1913b; American Nurses Association, 2009).

Conflict and Collaboration

Florence's Role
Conflict and Conflict Resolution
Florence understood that conflict is inevitable. She also appreciated the importance of resolving conflict positively. In her first nursing leadership position, she reported to a Council composed of a "Committee of Ladies" and a "Committee of Gentlemen" (Cook, 1913a, p. 133). The Ladies were difficult and Florence formed alliances within their group to accomplish her goals for patient care. Her cost-effective care won the support of her greatest opponent, who became her avid supporter throughout London (Cook, 1913a). This introduction to conflict in health care prepared Florence for even greater challenges in the Crimean War. Women had never worked in military hospitals, and many of the ladies who volunteered were not skilled nurses. Florence faced a monumental task—to find the right nurses, to manage them in a war zone, and to work collaboratively with the medical and military authorities there (Cook, 1913a). She understood that she would face military prejudice against women in war and medical jealousy against a woman in a position of authority in their hospitals. She realized that to succeed she must strictly adhere to rules, maintain firm discipline, and follow medical orders (Cook, 1913a). Some of the medical officers were resentful and placed obstacles in the way of "the Bird" as they called her (Cook, 1913a, p. 182). She never lost her temper and remained calm

at all times. In one ward, the junior medical officers were told to have nothing to do with her. She was patient and told her nurses "only to attend to patients in the wards of those surgeons who wished for our services, and she charged [them] never to do anything for the patients without the leave of the doctors" (Cook, 1913a, p. 182). Florence demonstrated tact and diplomacy along with self-restraint as her nurses' duties and wards varied based on the desire of the surgeons. She gradually won over skeptical physicians as they observed her efficiency and helpfulness. Even her most vociferous critic, Lieutenant-Colonel Anthony Sterling, had to acknowledge her power (Cook, 1913a). Many years later, the president of the College of Surgeons, a senior surgeon at St. Thomas' Hospital criticized the use of the Nightingale Fund to improve training for nurses (Cook, 1913b). Florence continued to quietly move forward with her school to make nursing a respected profession. Her success was illustrated in her May 23, 1873, address to nurses and probationers of the Nightingale School at St. Thomas' Hospital: "In the last ten years, thank God, numerous Training Schools for Nurses have grown up, resolved to unite in putting a stop to such a thing as drunken, immoral, and inefficient Nursing" (Nightingale, 2012, p. 46). Florence's approach to conflict management reflected her era, where English ladies were reserved and demure. Her strength lay in continuing to pursue her goals calmly and resolutely in the face of opposition (Cook, 1913a; Cook, 1913b).

Collaborating with Other Disciplines

Florence demonstrated exceptional collaboration skills throughout her life in interactions with diverse society members and groups. She had an uncanny ability to draw others to her and her causes. During her time at Scutari and the Crimea, Florence had powerful supporters in the government, the military, and the medical establishment (Cook, 1913a). Her earliest, staunchest supporter was Sidney Herbert, who facilitated her appointment as "Superintendent of the female nursing establishment in the English General Military Hospitals in Turkey" (Cook, 1913a, p. 155). He sent other letters to military and medical commanders and the Purveyor-General to elicit support for Florence and her nurses (Cook, 1913a). On her arrival, Florence collaborated with Dr. E. A. Parkes, the Superintendent of the Civil Military Hospital at Renkioi. Although she had no responsibility for the nursing care there, he regularly sought her advice and they developed a lifelong friendship (Cook, 1913a). The Commander, Lord Raglan, was totally supportive of Florence and her care for his wounded soldiers (Cook, 1913a). Many of the doctors welcomed Florence and her staff when they saw how efficient and effective she was in improving the patient care and cleanliness of the hospitals (Cook, 1913a). Her own nursing skills and compassion endeared her to the patients, while her willingness to teach endeared her to the orderlies (Cook, 1913a). The Senior Chaplain also became Florence's ally. In addition to supplying the needs of patients and hospitals, Florence also served as banker for officers at Scutari who entrusted her with their money rather than the Commissary or Purveyor (Cook, 1913a). Florence had connections with the Queen, her Court, and the war office that helped her influence the Sanitary Commission led by Dr. John Sutherland to reform military hospitals by sanitary engineering in 1855. Florence was passionate about reforming army hygiene and she collaborated with Dr. Sutherland on sanitary reforms for many years (Cook, 1913a). There are numerous examples of Florence's collaboration with Royals, government officials, commissions, statisticians, sanitary engineers, architects, and other experts during her life, resulting in improved health care and sanitation for civilian populations in England and abroad. She had a unique ability to involve these diverse professionals in partnership that ultimately transformed the lives of endangered communities (Cook, 1913a; Cook, 1913b).

The Nurse Manager's Role
Conflict and Conflict Resolution

You also know that conflict is inevitable and you realize that not all conflict is negative. Although nursing and health care have changed in the past 160 years, jealousy and prejudice still exist. The majority of nurses and nurse leaders continue to be women. Although men have been employed in nursing throughout history, their reputation in the early twentieth century was "drunk and incompetent" as female nurses were considered in the 1800s (O'Lynn, 2013, p. 33; Cook, 1913a). For example, let's say that you have been a male OR travel nurse for the past three years while you sought the perfect location and position for the rest of your nursing career. Now, you have found both. After extensive interviews, you are the first man to be nursing manager of Surgical Services in a 40-bed hospital on the New England seashore. In fact, you are the only man in management there except for the CEO. You are comfortable with conflict and approach it differently than your female counterparts. You are also getting used to a new organization, colleagues, co-workers, and community. That means there are multiple opportunities for conflict and conflict resolution in your new location. You also realize that diversity does not just include racial and ethnic minorities. In your new role and profession, you are also a minority by your gender (O'Lynn, 2013; Ives Erickson, Jones, & Ditomassi, 2013). As Florence prepared to enter Scutari, you also prepare to handle conflict as a nurse manager.

Your initial source of conflict is your director who is a micromanager. She wants to know what you are doing all the time and, after a couple of weeks, you find her incessant interruptions are adversely affecting your time management. You realize that you need to manage your boss' expectations if you will succeed in your new position. You set up a private meeting with her to confront the situation collaboratively and resolve potential conflict (Cloud, 2006). To avoid an adversarial situation, you focus on helping your boss succeed in her role so you can succeed in yours by setting clear expectations for communication. Your proactive willingness to support her enables both of you to establish effective guidelines for information about your professional activities that meet both of your needs (Cloud, 2006). She may always be a micromanager, but you both agree about which and when interactions occur for both of you to succeed.

Shortly after you begin work, one of your nurses, Tracey, stops in your office to complain about Dr. Lewis, an anesthesiologist. She says that he jokes through time-outs and considers them frivolous. She has tried talking with him privately and gotten nowhere. Since she scrubs for most of his cases, his behavior and lack of concern for patient safety distresses her. Other surgery RNs don't want to scrub on cases where he administers anesthetic for the same reason. You thank Tracey for her honesty and, after talking with other scrub nurses, you decide to observe one of his cases. You see that Tracey is right. Dr. Lewis' behavior during the time-out is exactly as she described. After the case, you speak with the surgeon to hear his perspective. He doesn't like Dr. Lewis' behavior, but doesn't think it is worth it to cross him because he is a skilled anesthetist. Then, you alert your director to the issue and brainstorm approaches with her. She recommends that you talk privately with Dr. Lewis about the dangers of wrong-site surgery that the time-out prevents (Guglielmi et al., 2014). You calmly stress to him that he is risking potential career-ending legal and financial implications if he is involved in a wrong-site surgery that could have been prevented by attention to a time-out (Guglielmi et al., 2014). No one has put it to him that way before. He has been amused by everyone's attention to the time-out, but never considered himself liable for anything but his duties as an anesthetist. Your statement shows that his actions do have consequences—potentially negative ones for him. You tell him that from now on there is zero tolerance for his previous behavior. He agrees to stop joking and listen to future time-outs. Of course, you also alert the Risk Manager and Chief of Surgical Services about your conversation and monitor Dr. Lewis' performance in the OR. After he has successfully participated in several time-outs, Tracey and the other scrub nurses thank him for being a valued team member to reinforce positive behavior. You also ensure that everyone in surgical services, including physicians, respects and maintains the culture of safety (Guglielmi et al., 2014). You now have demonstrated that you can successfully handle and resolve conflicts in your new workplace by staying calm and adhering to standards, much as Florence did in the Crimea (Cook, 1913a).

Collaborating with Other Disciplines

You have a title, Manager of Surgical Services, and formal authority within the organization. There is one power that you cannot be given, but must earn—respect. As you continue to settle in to your new role, you realize the importance of ensuring trust between you and your nurses so they are empowered to act autonomously. You spend time getting to know your staff, working with them, and seeing how you can support each of them. You serve as a role model for patient-focused behaviors in the unit as Florence did in Scutari (Cook, 1913a). You also build relationships with other healthcare team members. Once you have earned your team's trust and respect, you will have a unit that consistently provides quality patient care (American Academy of Nursing, 2010). They will also feel confident collaborating with physicians and other disciplines about patient care issues because they have observed you in action (Sasser, 2010).

Shortly after your arrival, the organization begins investigating a new system for charging surgical supplies, using a team-focused approach. This is a great opportunity to have your nurses and techs collaborate with central service, respiratory therapy, surgeons, anesthesiologists, information systems, finance and budgeting, and for organization leaders to review available options and participate in system selection. You stress to your unit representatives that everyone must work as a team to accomplish this task. Everyone at the table has something to offer and they must focus on the big picture and key issues (Gebauer & Lowman, 2008). It is exciting for you to witness their engagement in this process and the give-and-take between professionals results in a new charging product that meets everyone's needs. You know that this is only the beginning of ongoing engagement, accountability, and autonomy for your nurses through collaboration with multiple disciplines (Gebauer & Lowman, 2008). As Florence transformed the lives of endangered communities through collaboration, you and your staff can transform patients' lives in partnership with other professionals (Cook, 1913a; Cook, 1913b). There are many challenges ahead, but you look forward to them (and to being here a long time)!

Ethical Practice

Florence's Role
Commitment to the Patient

Florence's commitment to the patient permeated all her activities as a nurse. She provided physical care to those others avoided. She nursed cholera patients in London and spent up to eight hours on her knees bandaging wounds while reassuring wounded soldiers at Scutari. Florence tended to the sickest soldiers herself and one night she and one of her nurses cared for five men considered hopeless cases. The next morning they had improved enough to tolerate surgery (Cook, 1913a). She exemplified our Code of Ethics for Nurses by delivering care that respected patients' needs and values without bias (American Nurses Association, 2001). Her calming presence during her night rounds was described in a soldier's letter: "Before she came, there was cussin' and swearin', but after that it was holy as a church" (Cook, 1913a, p. 237). Florence recorded any dying soldier's last messages and wishes. Then, she forwarded these in letters to his loved ones at home. She also encouraged sick soldiers to write home and supplied paper and stamps. If they could not write, Florence, one of her nurses, or a volunteer wrote as they spoke (Cook, 1913a). Florence understood that "[t]he nurse's primary commitment is to the patient, whether an individual, family, group or community" (American Nurses Association, 2001, p. 9). Her *Notes on Nursing* reflects this, and she exemplified this in her later work to reform workhouse nursing and to institute district (community) nursing (Cook, 1913b). Florence personified the Provisions of our Code of Ethics for Nurses in a time when today's Code did not exist (American Nurses Association, 2001). She truly exemplified ethical practice in delivery of patient care.

Commitment to the Profession

Florence's commitment to the nursing profession was legendary. Her ethical practice demonstrated that a nurse owed the same duties to self that he or she accorded others: preserving self-respect, sustaining competence, continuing professional growth, expressing own moral point-of-view in practice, and maintaining integrity (American Nurses Association, 2001). Florence lived in an era when science was rapidly developing in health care. Her perspective that education and devotion to nursing were crucial for students and practicing nurses included scientific methods of providing care. She was aware that nurses had to remain competent and grow professionally every day if they, and the profession, were to advance (Cook, 1913a). To foster probationers' ethical and moral development, Florence required students in the Nightingale School to live on a new wing on an upper floor of St. Thomas' Hospital while they received technical training there (Cook, 1913a). A Matron closely supervised them and they met with the Chaplain twice a week (Cook, 1913a). She also played a significant role in preparing these future nurses by monitoring their progress, suggesting improvements, and encouraging them to embrace morality, self-respect, and integrity in their personal and professional lives (Nightingale, 2012). Florence's own words to her probationers on May 23, 1873, reveal her religious philosophy as well as her support for them and their chosen profession: "Without deep religious purpose how shallow a thing is Hospital life, which is, or ought to be, the most inspiring!" (Nightingale, 2012, p. 29). Florence also said,

> We are the more bound to watch strictly over ourselves; we have not less but more need of a high standard of duty and life in our Nursing; we must teach ourselves humility and modesty by becoming more aware of our own weakness and narrowness, and liability to mistake as Nurses and as Christians. Mere worldly success to any nobler, higher mind is not worth having. (Nightingale, 2012, p. 30)

Adherence to ethical principles guided Florence's life as well as her commitment to nursing and its future as a profession.

The Nurse Manager's Role
Commitment to the Patient

As a manager and a nurse, you must adhere to the content of the Code of Ethics for Nurses because it defines the values, goals, and duties of the profession (American Nurses Association, 2001). Your nurses must also practice based on these ethical standards when caring for patients. The Code must be easily accessible for future reference. You can keep a copy of the latest edition in a central location or ask for it to be put on your hospital's intranet. Whatever you decide, you need to have a conversation with your nurses about the content and importance of the Code for practicing nurses. Now, let's take a look at how they can use the provisions related to patient care in your medical unit.

The following two *Values in Action!* are very different, but demonstrate the fundamental ethical values and commitments of nurses to patients and families (American Nurses Association, 2001). As Florence embodied ethical practice in nursing care delivery, these examples validate that ethical practice in nursing care delivery is still active today.

Commitment to the Profession

Your must honor your ethical commitment to the nursing profession regardless of your role. However, as a nurse manager, you serve as a role model for nurses within your unit and organization by your leadership. Page 72 shows three examples from the Code of Ethics for Nurses (American Nurses Association, 2001).

Values in Action!

John Doe was just admitted from ED after he was found unconscious in an alley downtown, the victim of an apparent mugging. He has multiple bruises and abrasions as well as a concussion. He has no identification and his blood alcohol level was 0.8 on arrival. He is semi-conscious and slightly combative. Karen, a PCT and nursing student, tells Susan, the Charge Nurse, that he is probably "a homeless drunk." Susan informs her that every patient deserves respectful and compassionate care, including Mr. Doe. Karen apologizes and Susan helps her settle Mr. Doe into bed and clean his abrasions. Susan talks with the patient even though he is largely unresponsive. When he becomes agitated, Susan calmly strokes his hand and tries softly singing to him. He responds to her voice and slowly relaxes. Susan asks Karen if she can sit with this patient without judging him and his behavior. After getting an affirmative response, Susan tells his assigned nurse that she will monitor Mr. Doe during the rest of the shift. She ensures that Karen is providing safe care to Mr. Doe with attention to his rights as a patient. By the end of the shift, the patient is conscious and responsive. He now remembers his name and that he had a couple of drinks with friends last evening after work. Then, he decided to walk to his girlfriend's house a few blocks away. He was mugged on the way there and his wallet was taken. Karen asks to talk with Susan privately and apologizes for her initial reaction to the patient. Susan tells her that she has learned a valuable lesson with this patient. Often, first impressions are misleading, but even if he had been homeless and alcoholic, the nurse's duty is to the patient and the nurse's obligation is to protect his rights, health, and safety (American Nurses Association, 2001). Susan has used this opportunity as a learning experience for Karen about implementing the patient care Provisions of the *Code of Ethics for Nurses* (American Nurses Association, 2001).

Values in Action!

Henry has stage IV liver cancer and has been an inpatient on your unit many times during the past year. He has a partner, Bob, who has been with him for ten years. When he and Bob 'came out' to their families, both families severed ties with them. Henry knows that he is terminal and wants to stop treatment, but Bob is encouraging him to continue. You have developed a positive relationship with both men and stop on rounds to see how Henry is today. Henry is alone, tells you he is tired, and wants this to end. You ask if he and Bob have agreed on the decision to stop treatment. He believes Bob is holding out for a cure that is no longer possible. Bob comes in as you are speaking. You know that Henry has autonomy and self-determination to move to palliative care (American Nurses Association, 2001). You also know that this decision affects both men and that Bob must be able to support Henry's choice. You give them privacy for discussion and enable their spiritual advisor to collaborate with them as they soul-search this traumatic decision. After two days, they agree that palliative care is the correct action for Henry. You arrange for palliative care on your unit where both partners are supported throughout the dying process. You also ensure that follow-up care is available for Bob to help him deal with his loss. You have implemented the patient care provisions of the Code of Ethics for Nurses by providing compassionate and respectful care to both partners in this end-of-life scenario (American Nurses Association, 2001).

Example 1—Delegation and Accountability for Patient Care

Your nursing organization has policies and procedures for delegation by nurses. You must ensure that staff nurses delegate tasks appropriately to the person best suited for those tasks. They also must remember that they are accountable for nursing practice and patient care (American Nurses Association, 2001). You can reinforce appropriate delegation as you round on the unit and in conversation with nursing personnel.

Example 2—Improving the Healthcare Environment

You must maintain practice environments that support nurses in meeting their ethical obligations. These environments include working conditions, policies, procedures, job descriptions, job descriptions, disciplinary procedures, health and safety initiatives, grievance procedures, and compensation systems. As a nurse manager, you will be involved in many of these measures by participating in decision-making groups. You need to advocate for a culture that supports nurses to practice according to standards of care and treats them fairly (American Nurses Association, 2001).

Example 3—Duties Owed by the Nurse to Self

You have a responsibility to help your nurses preserve their self-respect, sustain competence, continue professional growth, express own moral point-of view in practice, and maintain integrity. As the manager, you engage nurses in opportunities for professional growth to increase their clinical competence. These opportunities may include continuing education, networking, self-study, formal education, and certification. You must treat all your nurses respectfully and encourage them to articulate their moral viewpoints even when they differ from others. You must also encourage your nurses to come to you if they are asked to do something that threatens their integrity and ability to be consistent with their professional and personal values. Such threats may include requests to withhold information, falsify a record, or lie to a patient. Verbal abuse from patients or co-workers cannot be tolerated (American Nurses Association, 2001). As Florence's commitment to nursing was based on ethical principles, your commitment to the profession must be predicated on the Code of Ethics for Nurses (American Nurses Association, 2001).

Focusing on Safety

Florence's Role

Environment of Care

The environment of care was vastly different in Florence's time. Civilian and military hospitals were not conducive to healing. After Kaiserwerth, which was plain, but clean, the Barrack Hospital at Scutari was horrendous (Cook, 1913a). Florence saw miles of wards with wooden cots no more than two feet apart with a 2 to 3 foot walkway in the middle. When there were too many wounded, Florence and her nurses had mattresses stuffed and put on the floor wherever there was room so the new wounded could be washed, bedded down, and have their wounds cleaned and dressed. Amputations were frequent, many of multiple limbs, and occurred in the same wards without even a screen until Florence provided one. Patients suffered from fevers, dysentery, and gangrene and the hospital was infested with lice and rats. In addition to lack of supplies, bedding, and clothing, the lack of sanitation was appalling. One of Florence's first acts was to have the floors scrubbed. Ventilation was poor and sewers under the floors were full of excrement. When the wind blew, sewer air came up the pipes of open latrines into the wards (Cook, 1913a). Besides focusing on cleanliness, Florence convinced the Sanitary Commission to accomplish sanitary engineering and resolve the drainage issues. This action resulted in a significant reduction of the death rate at the Barrack Hospital due to Florence's advocacy to improve the environment of care (Cook, 1913a). Florence also investigated the environment of care in civilian hospitals after returning home. She worked successfully for workhouse reform after finding that sick wards in city workhouses were unsanitary and overcrowded, with beds causing bedsores, deficiency of care supplies, dirty eating utensils, and inadequate cold food (Cook, 1913b). Hospitals also were built with corridors that limited ventilation combined with wards that had similar drainage issues and sewer smells as previously described (Cook, 1913a). Although these problems were not as intense as in the Crimea, Florence campaigned for the pavilion style of hospital construction to ensure adequate ventilation and space for the sick to recover (Nightingale, 1863). When she lost this battle over Netley Hospital, she managed to ensure that the corridor was wider, the wards had more window space, odd corners were removed, and ventilation was improved. Florence was a visionary whose recommendations about hospital construction are widely used in today's hospital construction projects (Cook, 1913a). She understood that the environment where care is delivered will positively or adversely affect the patient's safety and recovery.

Infection Prevention

Florence emphasized the importance of cleanliness and hand washing in preventing infection. We have already seen how she restored cleanliness and order in the wards at Scutari as well as ensuring that linens were washed in hot water (Cook, 1913a). Florence advocated hygiene to prevent mortality and saw mortality reduced after six months in the Crimea (Cook, 1913a). She cautioned nurses to keep patients clean by using hot, not cold, water. Her advice to them also included: "Every nurse ought to be careful to wash her hands very frequently during the day" (Nightingale, 1992, p. 53). Florence also addressed her probationers on April 28, 1876 about cleanliness and fresh air. "[T]here can be no pure air without cleanliness—Cleanliness is the only real Disinfectant. The least carelessness in not washing your hands between one bad case and another...may cost a life" (Nightingale, 2012, p. 119). She also advocated "isolation and extreme cleanliness" (Cook, 1913b, p. 197) for lying-in (maternity) hospitals, and provided plans for sanitary childbirth (Cook, 1913b). Florence's advocacy to prevent infection for patients, nurses, and native populations around the world is a tribute to her tenacity and focus on safety (Cook, 1913b).

The Nurse Manager's Role

Environment of Care

Your hospital and unit are very different from what Florence experienced in her lifetime. Even if your unit is not going to be remodeled, you still need to pay attention to the environment for patients, visitors, staff, and other healthcare team members. The delivery of patient care changes over time as new procedures and technologies are developed. You need to be proactive in assessing physical facilities to ensure a safe, effective setting for patients and nurses.

Your inpatient surgical unit has admitted several bariatric patients lately and you have two nurses on restricted duty from lifting injuries. There is also the potential for patient falls from this population. There is a designated lift on the adjacent wing, but nurses don't want to take the time to get the lift and set it up when patients want to move to a chair or go to the bathroom. You realize that ceiling lifts would be ideal, but there is no funding designated for them. You tell your nurses that they must use the available lift, but they believe the time spent in preparation will reduce the quality of patient care, particularly when the patient must use the bathroom or commode now. You meet with the safety officer and your director to address options. The safety officer suggests that a lift device be placed on your unit from another area where it has minimal use and the location be evaluated in 30 days. Your director will talk with the CNO about funding to put a ceiling lift in one of the patient rooms. You also order turning sheets to more easily move patients in bed. It won't totally solve the problem, but it is a start. You plan to request another ceiling lift in next year's Capital Equipment process. You meet with your nurses to determine a location for the portable lift and monitor that they actually are using it during the next 30 days. After that time, the manager of the 'loaner' unit says you can store the lift and they will borrow it if needed. The CNO can fund one ceiling lift now so you plan to schedule that room for bariatric patients. Your nurses like the lift being accessible quickly and are actually using it. Nurses are safely practicing their profession and providing safe patient care in the clinical environment (American Nurses Association, 2013a). Florence would be pleased.

Infection Prevention

Florence's focus on hand hygiene to prevent infection is applicable to today's nursing practice. You must monitor your unit to ensure that hand hygiene products and facilities are accessible to staff, patients, and visitors. You also must monitor staff compliance with hand hygiene practices as well as your own compliance. As the manager, you are a role model for professional behavior and this is one aspect of professional behavior. Infection prevention is an appropriate topic for unit meetings and Infection Surveillance Committee reports should be shared with staff members to monitor any trends. Look for a Champion on the unit to role model positive behaviors and 'encourage' colleagues to do the same. This does not have to be an RN, but other staff members must respect the Champion. Hand hygiene is an ongoing skill and positive feedback will encourage it to continue. You can even involve your patients and empower them to remind a caregiver to perform hand hygiene. That is especially helpful for visiting healthcare team members to the unit. Everyone must understand that hand hygiene protects healthcare workers as well as patients (World Health Organization, 2009).

Quality Improvement and Care Coordination

14

Florence's Role

Quality Improvement

Florence realized that quality improvement takes time. One example of this was her fight for workhouse reform in England. You saw in the previous chapter how terrible conditions were in those sick wards. The Poor Law Board made that observation in 1866 (Cook, 1913b). However, Florence's reform work to improve the quality of care in these facilities began in 1861. That year a philanthropist in Liverpool who was interested in establishing district nursing for the poor there approached her. The workhouse infirmary there needed a lady superintendent and trained nurses to replace the untrained, inefficient pauper nurses currently employed there. Florence selected Agnes Jones and sponsored her as she hired a staff and began to reform the facility. Florence carefully monitored the experiment's changes and success from 1861 to 1864 (Cook, 1913b). In 1864, she began communicating with the president of the Poor Law Board, since newspapers were inciting public opinion about the callous treatment of poor patients in workhouse wards. She appealed to the president's concern about preventing such scandals by such experiments as the Liverpool Workhouse Infirmary. Sensing his support, Florence began collecting the facts about all London infirmaries. Her approach was similar to quality improvement activities in today's hospitals. She developed a list of questions for use by the Poor Law inspector for the Metropolitan District. He issued the forms for completion in duplicate with one set returned to Florence for analysis. Florence knew that reform in administration and finance was required. Political changes in 1866 interfered and Florence continued her quality improvement journey with a Tory, rather than a Whig, government. A bill that she did not fully support started the legislative process. When it was adopted on March 29, 1867, significant reforms occurred for these workhouses. Florence decided that it was a beginning and the Act of 1867 became the foundation for quality improvements in medical relief under the Poor Law (Cook, 1913b). Florence deserved the credit for this significant legislation by influencing public opinion for workhouse reform. Her dedication to these reform efforts continued and resulted in employment of only trained nurses in workhouses by 1897 (Cook, 1913b). Florence's use of quality improvement principles resulted in successful legislation and, most of all, significant improvement in the care of poor people in these infirmaries.

Care Coordination
The best example of Florence's care coordination occurred in 1890 when she coordinated creation of "Health Missioners" for villages throughout England (Cook, 1913b, p. 384). County councils could tax and spend money on "Technical Education," which was broadly defined (Cook, 1913b, p. 383). They also received additional money from the Local Taxation Act of 1890 "Whiskey Money" (Cook, 1913b, p. 383). Florence wanted to use funds for "health at Home" and coordinated this with the chairman of the Technical Education Committee of North Bucks (Cook, 1913b, p. 383). She also coordinated with the health officer for the district to train ladies in classes to prepare them for this new role. He also provided a practicum for them in some of the villages. They accompanied him on rounds and he introduced them to village mothers and gave them advice on teaching villagers. Then, the ladies took an independent exam to test their knowledge. Those who passed completed a probationary period working with villagers and satisfactory performance resulted in obtaining certificates as Health Missioners. In 1892, the program was a success largely thanks to Florence's efforts. She recruited ladies, collected the best information about simple sanitary education, corresponded with other technical education committees, and sent a paper on rural hygiene to the Women Workers Conference in Leeds (November 1893) that is topical today (Cook, 1913b). Florence realized that care coordination is essential for lasting quality improvement to occur.

The Nurse Manager's Role

Quality Improvement

You have access to numerous quality improvement/process improvement tools and data in your daily work. These include unit quality dashboards, Clinical Process of Care Measures metrics, Clinical Outcome Measures metrics, voluntary turnover data, nursing hours per patient day (NHPPD), hospital consumer assessment of healthcare providers and systems (HCAHPS) patient satisfaction data, National Database of Nursing Quality Indicators (NDNQI) data, and specific organization QI/PI measures (Centers for Medicare and Medicaid Services, 2013b; Centers for Medicare and Medicaid Services, 2013a; National Quality Forum, 2004). One increasing metric that is disturbing to you is the number of seclusions for violent behavior in your emergency department (ED). This is reflected in nursing injuries from combative patients. You need a quality improvement initiative to address this issue by initiating practice changes that will minimize this number and protect patients and staff. This goal is in alignment with the Standards of Professional Performance for Nursing Administration (American Nurses Association, 2009, p. 35). You meet with your department's quality coordinator to assess available resources for de-escalation of agitated behavior (Richmond et al., 2012). As Florence realized in her workhouse example, you know that data is important to determine the results of change. You have baseline data on your monthly quality reports. Now, you form a PI team, including your CNS, quality coordinator, and staff representatives from nursing and support departments, like security. After reviewing the literature, a verbal de-escalation approach is trialed. It is important that the physical space is safe and staff members are trained and able to work with these patients. An adequate number of trained staff members must be available and objective scales are used to assess agitation. Clinicians must self-monitor and safely approach the patient (Richmond et al., 2012). Domains of de-escalation also help clinicians care for agitated patients (Richmond et al., 2012, p. 20). After the trial, the team reviews the latest quality data about seclusions. There has been a significant reduction since the initiation of the trial. The improved process has also reduced nursing injuries on the unit. This change in nursing practice, based on a quality improvement project, has accomplished the desired results for your patients and staff, as Florence's workhouse reform did in the nineteenth century in England (Cook, 1913b; American Nurses Association, 2009).

Care Coordination

You are the nurse manager on a geriatric unit and Linda, one of your nurses, comes to you with a concern. Mr. Porter, an 89-year-old with diabetes, right below the knee amputation, glaucoma, and hypertension, is ready for discharge to an assisted care facility. However, he wants to go home where he lives alone. He was widowed seven years ago and has one son who lives in another state. There are no other relatives in the area. He is adamant about going home. You meet with the patient and he understands that he has multiple health issues. His glaucoma is stable and the hypertension is under control. The amputation occurred three years ago and his home is equipped for wheelchair access. He was hospitalized this time because a case of flu "got my sugar out of whack." He has a neighbor (age 75) who "looks out for me." After talking with Mr. Porter, you contact his son 400 miles away. He is not surprised because his father loves the house and has told him, "They'll have to carry me out." He is willing to come if needed or take his father home with him if he will consent. Mr. Porter says 'no' to both. You and Linda decide to hold a care coordination conference and seek input from other members of the healthcare team. You and Linda meet with Mr. Porter's primary care physician, social worker, dietician, physical therapist, home care nurse, clinical nurse specialist, and cardiology nurse practitioner. After everyone discusses the benefits of a transfer to assisted care for Mr. Porter, you steer the conversation to "How can we ensure his safety in his home?" That discussion is intense, but in the end, a plan is in place for Mr. Porter to go home with support from home health, social work, a nutritionist, physical therapy using the medical home concept with his primary care physician coordinating all care activities (AHRQ Care Coordination, 2014). He comes to the table for review of the care plan post-discharge. Mr. Porter agrees and returns to his home with this interdisciplinary support. A week later, you see Mr. Porter's physician on rounds and ask how he is doing. He is doing fine at home and getting lots of attention. You both smile and are pleased that care coordination has worked to Mr. Porter's benefit (AHRQ Care Coordination, 2014). You have demonstrated Florence's realization that care coordination is essential for lasting quality improvement to occur.

The Importance of Evidence and Research in Daily Practice

Florence's Role

Evidence in Practice

Florence was passionate about statistics and their practical uses. She was elected a member of the Statistical Society in 1858 and her focus was hospital statistics (Cook, 1913a). There was no common standard and each hospital used its own nomenclature and classification of diseases. With support from a leading statistician and friendly doctors, Florence created a standard list of classes and orders of diseases and model hospital statistical forms to determine accurate mortality rates in different hospitals and mortality from diseases and injuries for various age groups (Cook, 1913a). The value of treatments and special operations could be statistically proven and the sanitary condition of the hospital could be determined (Cook, 1913a). Several hospitals adopted her forms and she and the statistician studied the results. He was one of the general secretaries of the International Statistical Congress, which met in London in the summer of 1860. Florence's forms were the major topic of discussion. The Congress voted to present her forms to each government represented there. (Cook, 1913a). She did not succeed in the adoption of her forms by every English hospital, but continued to press the government to publish more statistical data. She encouraged additional questions in the census of 1861 to collect statistical data for sanitary improvements. Although this change was not made,

Florence's request was ahead of her time and additional questions were finally added to future census forms (Cook, 1913a). These are only a few examples of her use of evidence to improve practice in England and other countries.

Research in Practice

Florence did significant research on sanitation issues in India, which began with the development of a Royal Sanitary Commission for the Armies in India. Florence had spent two years asking Lord Stanley for a Commission and it was created in 1859. Florence analyzed mortality statistics of the Indian Army and noted that neglect of sanitary precautions resulted in the deaths of British soldiers stationed there (Cook, 1913b). Although she was not a member of the Commission, Florence performed the research it used in its deliberations and final report. She immediately collected, prepared, and processed evidence for the Commission. She and a leading statistician began working on ten years of Army mortality and illness statistics. In 1863, the Indian Sanitary Commission released a 2028-page report in small print. The report contained 23 pages written by Florence and contained illustrations of Indian hospitals and barracks as well as native customs related to water supply and drainage (Cook, 1913b). Her written *Observations* were circulated separately with the report, with one copy sent to the Queen (Cook, 1913b, p. 25). Florence's research on India and its sanitation was vast and gave the impression that she actually went there, although she never did. It is impressive that she did this research and work for the Commission at a time when she was bedridden, could only have visitors, and write while lying in bed (Cook, 1913b). Florence's dedication to this cause empowered her to see this study through to the end.

The Nurse Manager's Role

Evidence in Practice

You are the nurse manager in the ICU (Intensive Care Unit). Eric, one of your staff nurses just returned from NTI (National Teaching Institute and Critical Care Exposition) and he is excited (AACN home page, n.d.). He attended a session about the importance of mobility for critical care patients and wants to see if evidence will support this for patients in your unit. You connect Eric with the hospital librarian and they perform a literature search. Eric returns with evidence that early ambulation and physical therapy are beneficial to the recovery of critical care patients (Adler & Malone, 2012). You and Eric talk with physical therapists, who are interested in the benefits to patients from physical therapy—improved activities of daily living, better muscle strength, and potential for reduced length of stay in ICU. Once you have their support, you both prepare a presentation for a unit meeting and gain the backing of the staff nurses to try this approach. Then, you and Eric meet with the Critical Care Leadership team, including the Chief of Service, and present a proposal to implement an early ambulation program in the ICU on a trial basis. There is some initial reluctance, but they decide to go ahead with the trial. You and Eric plan careful monitoring during the trial period to address safety issues and potential for adverse events as well as observed benefits to patients from early ambulation. Eric reviews statistical data about this practice change and evidence obtained during the trial. One patient experienced a significant increase in heart rate and respiratory rate during a therapy session. Another patient was accidently extubated during ambulation. The rest of the patients gained muscle strength by measurement and their movement improved from sitting to standing prior to transfer from ICU. The Step-down unit staff confirmed after transfer that these patients demonstrated improved mobility in bed and during transfers (Adler & Malone, 2012). Now, early ambulation and physical therapy are approved protocols for your unit. The hospital's Quality Board recognized Eric for his idea and use of evidence in practice as the International Statistical Congress recognized Florence for hers.

Research in Practice

You are the nurse manager of your hospital's Neonatal Intensive Care Unit (NICU). Today, the CNO asked for you and your director to meet with him. Erin James, a doctoral nursing student who is a per diem employee in ED, joins you to discuss her research proposal about job stress in NICU nurses. She has met with the Research Council about her research design and received their endorsement. She is applying to the Institutional Review Board (IRB) as an exempt study. Erin has copies of her proposal and her survey tool for each of you to review. Then, she would like to meet with your nurses to discuss her proposal and seek volunteers from the unit. You tell her you will contact her after reviewing her materials to discuss any questions and plan next steps.

When you return to your office, you review Erin's research design and process. She has done a comprehensive literature review of her research topic and has a well-developed hypothesis. Her research design is appropriate and she is obtaining required approvals from the IRB and hospital review panels. Erin's survey tool has been previously tested for reliability and validity and her data collection processes are appropriate for the study. Her data analysis process is comprehensive (Association for Nursing Professional Development, 2013). You are very impressed with her study and the topic intrigues you. NICU nurses nurture stressed families as well as premature infants. The emotional toll on the nurse can be great enough to result in burnout and transfer from the NICU (Cricco-Lizza, 2014). You are very interested in her results to implement interventions that will positively impact nurse job satisfaction, retention, and, most of all, consistent delivery of quality patient and family care (Cricco-Lizza, 2014). Erin obtains her IRB approval and you invite her to meet with the NICU nurses. A few are not interested in participating, but the majority of nurses want to be involved. Eight months later, Erin presents her results and you have some interventions that can help your nurses, including recognition and support for their emotional involvement with families (Cricco-Lizza, 2014). Erin's research is making a difference in your unit as Florence's research did in reducing mortality in India.

Transforming the Future of Nursing

16

Now, you know what a remarkable leader Florence Nightingale was and how relevant she is to today's nursing practice. Since you and Florence are comfortable with each other, it's time to contemplate the future for nurse leaders and the profession with her support. In the beginning, you examined the regulatory, quality, and reimbursement issues impacting today's healthcare scene, an alphabet soup of changes—VBP, HCAHPS, SCIP, CLABSI, CAUTI, HAPU, and VAP with more to come (Centers for Medicare and Medicaid Services, 2013b; Centers for Medicare and Medicaid Services, 2013a; National Quality Forum, 2004). The Institute of Medicine (IOM) Report is the current blueprint for the future of health care and nursing (Institute of Medicine, 2011). Nurses have an unprecedented opportunity to influence the future of health care in the United States. Let's look at how we can get there.

Education

Florence contended with uneducated, intoxicated women functioning as 'nurses' to the detriment of patients and the reputation of nursing. She devoted countless years and energy to provide education for nurses that would ensure quality patient care (Cook, 1913a; Cook, 1913b). Nurses today cannot stop learning just because they are licensed and working. As Florence said to the students of the Nightingale School,

> *For us who Nurse, our Nursing is a thing, which, unless we are making progress every year, every month, every week, take my word for it, we are going back. The more experience we gain the more progress we can make. The progress you make in your year's training with us is as nothing to what you must make every year after your year's training is over.* (Nightingale, 2012, p. 1)

If you substitute 'initial nursing education' for 'year's training,' Florence's statement is applicable to current and future nurses. Today, there is still conflict within the nursing profession about the level of education required to practice as a registered nurse. Most professions have a specified entry level to remain on a par with other professions requiring as much as six to eight years of formal education. Many healthcare organizations support the IOM's recommendations that 80% of nurses hold BSN or higher degrees by 2020 and that the numbers of doctoral-prepared nurses in the United States double. The Institute's report stated that Associate Degree Nurses (ADNs) are essential in the current healthcare delivery system, but recommended that additional formal education will position nurses to provide highly skilled care to complex and aging populations both within acute care and in the community (Institute of Medicine, 2011). The Magnet Recognition Program supports this move to greater formal nursing education in its 2014 Magnet Application Manual, which requires "[a]n action plan that includes a target and demonstrates evidence of progress toward 80% of registered nurses obtaining a baccalaureate or graduate degree in nursing by 2020" (American Nurses Credentialing Center, 2014, p. 27). Beyond formal education, Florence also advocated lifelong learning for nurses (Nightingale, 2012). Health care continuously changes as new advances occur in technology, pharmacology, and treatment options. It is imperative for nurses to read professional literature, attend continuing education offerings, and seek certification in their clinical specialties to enhance and validate their knowledge and skills in clinical practice (American Academy of Nursing, 2010).

The Nurse Manager's Role

What is your role in the educational future of nursing? You need to be a role model for supporting education, both formal and informal, for your staff and others in your organization. That means seeking and attaining an advanced degree yourself. It also means sharing positive feedback with others about education and the knowledge you are obtaining. You must:

- Support other nurses or those who want to become nurses with information about available programs and financial aid. Nursing education is expensive and many nurses who would love to have a BSN or MSN can't afford the financial cost without additional support;

- Know what scholarships, loans, and grants are out there;
- Get involved in initiatives to increase tuition assistance for employees as well as conference/continuing education funding; and
- Encourage gender and ethnic diversity in nursing education and practice. Nursing education and its practitioners must reflect the race, ethnicity, and gender profile of the community served (Ives Erickson, Jones, & Ditomassi, 2013).

If your organization doesn't have certification reimbursement, pursue it with your leaders and your hospital foundation. As a nurse manager, you are a leader and that is true for both formal and continuing nursing education. If a staff nurse is in a BSN program and must complete an eight-hour clinical experience weekly, you can work with the person to flex their schedule to meet the needs of the patients, the unit, and the employee's education. As a leader, you know your staff, their needs, strengths, and interests. Support their professional growth by facilitating their participation in continuing education activities that will increase their knowledge, skills, competencies, and decision-making abilities (Association for Nursing Professional Development, 2013). Lifelong learning must not just be a goal. It must be a daily reality in the future of nursing in the 21st century. You are a catalyst to sustain this reality so nursing can achieve transformative changes in health care.

Practice

Nursing practice in Florence's time was limited in scope. Most nurses were employed in workhouses or hospitals. Florence devoted her *Notes on Nursing* to how nursing should be practiced in hospitals and homes (Nightingale, 1992). She was a proponent of district (community) nursing and she was the first to introduce the concept of "nursing the well" (Nightingale, 1992, p. 6). Today, caring for "the well" is accepted in clinics and community practice environments. Prevention of disease and illness in these settings is a distinct role for Advanced Practice Registered Nurses (APRNs) with implications for future practice (Institute of Medicine, 2011). As healthcare costs continue to rise, these practitioners will play a key role in facilitating positive health behaviors for this population, resulting in cost reduction (Institute of Medicine, 2011). Transitioning primary care practices into patient-centered medical homes is in its infancy, but has promise for reducing hospital admission and healthcare costs. It also enables nurse practitioners to play a significant role in patient education and compliance (Institute of Medicine, 2011). As you can see, the practice field is diversifying for nurses, although there still will be a need for hospital-based nurses. Their roles will also transform in the future. As advanced practice nurses' roles in the community evolve, Clinical Nurse Leaders (Jeffers & Astroth, 2013) and Clinical Nurse Specialists are two roles that healthcare systems in the future will utilize to coordinate the continuum of care. Both advanced practice roles focus on integrated delivery services to achieve high-quality, cost-effective care (Ives Erickson, Jones, & Ditomassi, 2013; Jeffers & Astroth, 2013). Their collaboration with the Nurse Manager will benefit staff as well as patients in acute care settings.

The Nurse Manager's Role
You also must confront scope-of-practice issues for today's nurses (Institute of Medicine, 2011). Nursing requires practice changes to thrive in years to come. Nurses must use evidence and research in daily practice and stay alert to changes in reimbursement, quality, and regulatory issues that influence nurses' clinical practice. Nurse-sensitive indicators are opportunities for nurses to excel in acute care settings. You need to ensure that the nurses are knowledgeable about these indicators and their role in meeting them. As a nurse manager, you are responsible for marketing the excellence of your nurses in meeting indicators that affect the hospital's bottom line in reimbursement (Centers for Medicare and Medicaid Services, 2013b; National Quality Forum, 2004). Collaboration with Clinical Nurse Leaders and Clinical Nurse Specialists is vital for patient care. You must differentiate between these roles and establish a cohesive partnership to achieve unit nursing initiatives and organization goals (Edwardson & Irvin, 2013). You must involve your nursing team in this partnership because they are integral to its success. Two-way communication and follow-up are essential when implementing practice changes for the future (Edwardson & Irvin, 2013). Nurses must be armed with knowledge of evidence and research findings, clinical expertise, dedication to quality patient care, and your support to thrive in a changing practice climate. This is an exciting time for nurses, as they become leaders in health care, much as Florence did when she founded the modern nursing profession (Cook, 1913a; Cook, 1913b).

Influence
Florence's influence on health care was legendary. Besides founding the modern nursing profession, she was a recognized expert in numerous aspects of health care from sanitation to hospital construction (Cook, 1913a; Cook, 1913b). Today's nurses also influence the future of health care by their practice. As nurses move into new healthcare settings, their influence spreads. Their focus on outcomes and process improvement makes them invaluable providers (Ewoldt, 2014). It is now obvious that clinical knowledge is no longer enough to

thrive. Although clinical skills were important to Florence, she had the political savvy to deal proactively with multiple audiences and succeed in reaching her goals (Cook, 1913a; Cook, 1913b). Today's nurses must do the same.

The Nurse Manager's Role

You need to be politically savvy to help your nurses succeed. You may consider organizational politics negative, but they are far from that (Gentry & Brittain Leslie, 2012). You are learning your new role and navigating organizational politics is part of your role. Remember that you are accountable for the success or failure of your unit, your team, and nursing in your organization. You will have courses available to you on financial and personnel management, but most organizations don't educate new managers on the vital topic of political savvy. Politics is normal behavior and can be a win-win situation for everyone involved. You use your interpersonal skills and behaviors to be an effective leader. Political savvy doesn't mean promoting yourself at the expense of others. It can mean being genuine and positive by developing diverse networks and relationships that enable you to understand others at work and influence them as Florence did to reinforce professional and organizational objectives (Gentry & Brittain Leslie, 2012). This is your opportunity to positively persuade others that nurses are major players in the healthcare environment now and in the future.

Partnership

Florence formed unlikely partnerships over the years. Her relationship with prominent physicians helped her achieve her goal of trained nurses. Several of these men also partnered with the School's Matron to teach the students about disease processes and patient care (Cook, 1913a). Not all physicians were positive about Florence's decision to advance nursing education. Some of them felt that reform was not needed in nursing care. Nurses did what they were told and that was sufficient. It turned out that the current supply of nurses was not adequate to properly care for patients (Cook, 1913a). Today, the domination of patient care by physicians is receding, although some physicians are still opposed to the emergence of APRNs in decision-making roles at the point of care in the community (Institute of Medicine, 2011; Ives Erickson, Jones, & Ditomassi, 2013). Today's nurses must elicit physician support, as Florence did, to guarantee a healthcare future where nurses practice "to the full extent of their education, skills and competencies" (Institute of Medicine, 2011, p. 27-28). They must partner with physicians to improve patient care by collaboration and communication (Ives Erickson, Jones, & Ditomassi, 2013). This is a challenge and opportunity that must be met. Both roles are distinct and complementary. Each is also essential to navigate the complexities of patient care. A team approach with an attitude of mutual respect will result in collective action for the benefit of the most important person on the healthcare team now and in the future—the patient. Florence would heartily endorse this and add that careful nursing observation and assessment must be shared with the doctor to ensure an appropriate plan of care for the patient (Nightingale, 1992).

Both disciplines must include the patient as a participant in his or her care processes. Florence never lost sight of the importance of the patient—sick or well (Nightingale, 1992). Neither can we and other healthcare team members. The patient deserves no less.

The Nurse Manager's Role

Regardless of your care setting, you must facilitate partnerships between health professionals to improve patient care. Your own communication skills must be exceptional. You must role model collegial behavior for your team members. You must be confident in initiating crucial conversations to confront teamwork issues that may result in patient safety deficits or lapses in quality (Patterson et al., 2013). That includes relationships with physicians. If a physician doesn't perform hand hygiene before touching the patient, he or she puts that patient at risk. Often, the patient won't complain and sometimes nurses will ignore this behavior too. It is easier to avoid confrontation, but in health care, it is necessary (Patterson et al., 2013). Your communication must be clear and consistent as well as setting clear expectations for performance (Patterson et al., 2013). You must learn to approach the conversation with honesty and respect without alienating the other person. This won't be easy at first, but developing self-confidence in your skills will build, rather than weaken, relationships (Patterson et al., 2013). This is another aspect of your performance that must be cultivated. As with political savvy, crucial conversations are vital for partnerships that uphold patient safety and quality now and in the future. Florence successfully managed numerous crucial conversations with partners to resolution during her career (Cook, 1913a; Cook, 1913b). Now, it's your turn!

The future of nursing is up to you and your contemporaries. For nurses to thrive in a healthcare environment that will become increasingly complex will require:

- Lifelong learning through formal and continuing education;
- Ability to implement practice changes rapidly and well;
- Focus on outcomes and process improvement to influence the direction of health care; and
- Partnership with other disciplines, especially physicians, to improve patient care through communication and collaboration.

Last but by no means least, the patient must be at the center of health care. They are the reason we all come to work every day. If we remember that, we will navigate the waters of our healthcare environment as Florence navigated the waters of hers when she created the modern profession of nursing (Cook, 1913a; Cook, 1913b).

A Parting Word

Enjoy the challenges and opportunities of your new role and make Florence proud! You are the future that she dreamed about 160 years ago. She will always be your mentor as she mentored so many before you. Take advantage of every learning opportunity and, as you grow in your role and experience, always mentor others. That is your true legacy!

Congratulations and best wishes!

Index